You Don't Have to Die

You Don't

Have to

Die

One Family's Guide to

Surviving

Childhood Cancer

GERALYN AND CRAIG GAES
AND PHILIP BASHE

VILLARD BOOKS • NEW YORK • 1992

Villard Books is a registered trademark
of Random House, Inc.

Portions of this book have been adapted from the *USP
DI, Volume II, Advice for the Patient.* Copyright, the United
States Pharmacopeial Convention, Inc. Permission
granted. For additional information regarding the drugs
discussed in this book, copies of the *USP DI* can be
ordered from the USPC by calling (800) 227-8772.

Library of Congress Cataloging-in-Publication Data

Gaes, Geralyn.
You don't have to die: one family's guide to surviving childhood
cancer / Geralyn and Craig Gaes, Philip Bashe.
p.   cm.
ISBN 0-679-40300-0
1. Tumors in children. I. Gaes, Craig. II. Bashe, Philip.
III. Title.
RC281.C4G33   1992   91-51040
362.1′9699′442—dc20

9 8 7 6 5 4 3 2
First Edition

The text of this book is set in Baskerville.

So many people, both family and friends, helped us to piece our lives back together during our son Jason's illness. We dedicate this book to all of you. May its message of hope comfort those who read it, the same way that your love, friendship, and support have comforted us.

PREFACE

"If I am to be honest, I have to tell you . . . probably yes."

Years have passed, yet I can still hear those words, the doctor's grave tone, his hesitation before answering. The setting, too, remains vividly etched in my memory: My husband, Craig, and I sitting in a brightly sunlit consultation room at the Mayo Clinic. A children's-cancer specialist opposite us delivering as compassionately as possible the devastating news that our six-year-old son has a particularly deadly form of advanced cancer. Craig and I looking at each other in shock, then me asking tearfully, "Is Jason going to die?" Followed by the doctor's somber reply.

But our son didn't die. Two grueling years of intensive chemotherapy, radiation, and surgery—not to mention our flooding heaven with prayers—saved his life. Today Jason is a healthy, active teenager, a loyal Dan Marino and Larry Bird fan who rattles the walls of our home with rock music. He is also an author, of *My Book for Kids with Cansur*. (The title's misspelling was as close as he could come at the time.) Jason wrote it toward the end of his medical treatment, when he seemed well on the way to recovery.

I remember the two of us curled up on a sofa one afternoon flipping through a children's book about cancer, written by a young patient. As in several others we'd read together on the subject, at story's end the little boy died. "What a terrible book!" Jason fumed. "Why do they always write books and make movies and stuff about kids who die? Didn't they ever hear about somebody like me, who had cancer and grew up and lived? Why don't they write a book about that?"

Stuck for an answer, I suggested, "Maybe you ought to write your own book, Jason," never dreaming that he actually would.

"Well," he said with a huff, "maybe I ought to."

Several months later I was washing dishes when Jason bounded into the kitchen. "Here it is," he said as he casually handed me his "book," scrawled in a yellow spiral notebook. I admit, I'd expected some cutesy, silly little thing; nothing too profound. But as I turned the pages, tears streamed down my face. "If you get cansur, don't be scared," my son advised, " 'cause lots of people get over having cansur and grow up without dying." It was remarkable to me that a child could possess such insight about a disease many adults struggle to understand.

That night I gave it to my husband to read. Closing the cover, Craig wondered aloud, "Wouldn't it be something if we could get this into the hands of other mothers and fathers who are just starting down the path we're finishing up?" If our son's surviving cancer had taught us any lesson, it was that nothing is impossible. *My Book for Kids with Cansur,* illustrated by Jason's older brother, Adam, and Jason's twin, Tim, was published in 1987. Since then he has regularly received phone calls from young cancer patients all over the world who've found comfort in his message of hope.

Craig and I were moved to write about our family's experience out of the same frustration as Jason's. After he was diagnosed with Burkitt's lymphoma in 1984, we desperately pored through every book we could find on pediatric cancer. Though informative, most had the same shortcomings. They described in cold, clinical jargon what cancer is and printed neat statistical charts illustrating whom it strikes and so forth. But none of them conveyed *what it's like* when a child—your child—has cancer. Few resources we came across even mentioned, much less adequately prepared us for, the emotional upheavals and the unpredictable fears and feelings this crisis brings to bear on your entire family.

Another thing we found: book after book, article after article seemed to deify kids with cancer and their families, leaving the unsettling impression that the disease afflicted only special, extraordinary, heroic people. Well, when our family's world collapsed that day in the Mayo Clinic, neither Craig nor I felt particularly special. Certainly not extraordinary. And never heroic. Instead we felt much the same way you probably do right now if a child you know has cancer: scared and utterly helpless.

I suppose it's natural for parents to avoid thinking the unthinkable.

Who imagines that their home will be invaded and their child abducted by this vicious intruder? Certainly I didn't. Children's cancer, I thought, happens only to those wonderful, strong women canonized in *Ladies' Home Journal.* At the time of Jason's diagnosis I had never known anyone, adult or child, with cancer. I was a housewife and mother of four, one an infant daughter; Craig, a hardworking husband and father. We were a typical, close-knit family from rural Worthington, Minnesota. Our son's sickness crashed into our lives like a flaming meteor through the roof of our cozy home. To say we felt unprepared and overwhelmed is an understatement.

But you'd be amazed at your resiliency when your child's welfare is at stake. I love it when people say to me now, "Gee, Geralyn, you're such a strong person. I could never survive something like that." Of course they could. As parents you do whatever you have to for your ailing child. *You don't have any choice!* Our family's story is by no means one of heroism, just of human beings' remarkable ability to adapt and survive.

If there was one mistake my husband and I made, it was not realizing how a child's cancer impacts on every family member, and that each has his or her own capacity to cope. Relatives, friends, teachers, and co-workers all feel the profound effects of a youngster's catastrophic illness. To provide a full-family perspective, we've incorporated in this book the thoughts and feelings of Jason, his brothers, Adam and Tim, and his three surviving grandparents. As you'll see, not everyone reacts the same way, and a surprising number of us found ourselves responding in ways we'd never have imagined.

Craig and I were once in the position you may be in now: looking wistfully at your sick child and fearing you won't get to see him grow up. We sincerely hope that by reliving our experience as it unfolded and sharing what we learned, we can help other parents to meet a young patient's needs, their family's needs and, not to be overlooked, their own needs.

With that said, while we've intended *You Don't Have to Die* to provide practical advice and support in clear, straightforward language, we must stress that each case of cancer is unique. Some patients respond to treatment; others, tragically, do not. Nor do we want to diminish the gravity of pediatric cancer, which claimed an estimated 1,600 young lives in 1990, more than any other disease.

However, cancer researchers have made enormous and rapid progress, especially in the field of childhood cancers. Had Jason been stricken twenty years earlier, he almost certainly would have died within a matter of weeks. In the mid-1960s only one in five kids survived cancer, as opposed to one in three by the mid-1980s. Like most parents of children with cancer two decades before, we would have been gently advised to prepare for our son's imminent death. Today's cure rate has reached an all-time high of more than two in three, with recent medical advances further supporting hopes for a child's recovery.

Cancer afflicts more youngsters than ever before, the number of cases rising 15 percent from 1989 to 1990 alone. That means more families will endure the protracted treatment and recovery, an uncertain time of seesawing emotions. Household routines are disrupted, finances devoured, marriages severely tested, and the entire family's future, for all intents and purposes, suspended.

It takes love and faith to emerge from such an experience intact, and it's not easy. But I must tell you that when this happened to Jason and our family, I thought our lives would always center around his disease and could never, ever be pieced back together again. But as time passed, that proved not to be the case. We hope readers will look at us, see how our lives have evolved, and realize that they are not alone. People do withstand this crisis. There *can* be life after children's cancer. We are proof of that.

Geralyn Gaes
1992

ACKNOWLEDGMENTS

The authors would like to thank the following for providing print materials and/or assistance: AirLifeline; AMC Cancer Research Center; American Association of Blood Banks; American Cancer Society; American College of Surgeons; American Institute for Cancer Research; American Society of Clinical Oncologists; Association for the Care of Children's Health; Association for Research of Childhood Cancer, Inc.; Cancer Care, Inc.; Candlelighters Childhood Cancer Foundation; CanHelp; Center for Attitudinal Healing; Centers for Disease Control; Children's Cancer Research Institute; Children's Hospice International; Children's Oncology Camps of America, Inc.; Compassionate Friends; Corporate Angel Network; Department of Health and Human Services, Social Security Administration; Epidemiology Resources, Inc.; Foundation for Advancement in Cancer Therapies.

Also: Hereditary Cancer Institute at Creighton University School of Medicine, Omaha, Nebraska; International Association of Cancer Victims and Friends; Leukemia Society of America, Inc.; Lineberger Cancer Research Center, School of Medicine at the University of North Carolina at Chapel Hill; Make Today Count; Mayo Clinic; Minnesota Department of Health; Nassau County Department of Health; National Cancer Center; National Cancer Institute, Office of Cancer Communications; National Center for Education in Maternal and Children's Health; National Coalition for Cancer Survivorship; National Foundation for Cancer Research; New York State Insurance Department; Kenneth J. Norris Jr. Cancer Hospital, Los Angeles, California; R. A. Bloch Cancer Foundation; Ronald McDonald House; Skin Cancer Foundation; and the United States Pharmacopeial Convention.

We are especially grateful to Dr. Gerald Gilchrist, Dr. Omer Burgert, Dr. William Smithson, Dr. Paula Schomberg, Donna Betcher and Ginny Rissmiller of the Mayo Clinic, and Dr. Karen Bringelsen for their kind cooperation and generosity of time; Mary Ellen Landwehr of the Mayo Clinic News Bureau; Florence S. Antoine of the National Cancer Institute media office; Stacy Charney of the American Cancer Society media office; Mrs. Susan Arleo; filmmaker Bill Guttentag; our editor, Diane Reverand; her assistant, Amy Einhorn; copy editor Daia Gerson; agent Suzanne Gluck of International Creative Management; and her assistant, Kate Renko.

Philip Bashe would like to separately thank agent Sarah Lazin; her assistant, Laura Nolan; agent Jed Mattes; Leila Barconey; Rochelle and Robert Bashe; the late Evelyn Bashe; and, as always, Patty Romanowski Bashe.

CONTENTS

You Don't Have to Die

CHAPTER ONE

"WHAT WE FOUND WAS A MALIGNANCY"

Biopsies • Breaking the News to Your Child and Other Family Members

Our lives are marked by anniversaries: births, graduations, weddings. Just as navigators at sea fix on the stars to determine their position, observing those personal chronological landmarks helps us to chart our course through life. But when a child falls prey to cancer, all other signposts recede into the distance. Our son, Jason, then six, was diagnosed with the disease on Thursday, June 28, 1984. For the next five years that date became a benchmark of life and death against which we measured everything.

Cancer can develop undetected for many months, yet it steals up on you like a thief in the night. Our family's ordeal began innocently enough one gloriously sunny Tuesday morning. My husband, four young children, and I were staying over at his mother's home in Storm Lake, Iowa. We planned to leave that afternoon for a summer vacation at Worlds of Fun, a Kansas amusement park the kids had been clamoring to visit.

Jason, an early riser, hopped out of bed around daybreak. Only his Uncle Terry, who is deaf, was up. The two began playing around with a flashlight, Jason shining it in Terry's eyes and ears. Then his uncle took the flashlight, joking, "Let me see if you've got any cavities."

Jason obediently opened his mouth. Terry immediately noticed an ugly bump about the size of a grape hanging from our son's upper gum. Aiming the beam closer, he saw it was blackish in color. When I padded downstairs to fetch myself a cup of coffee, Terry pointed it out to me.

Since the bump sat where Jason's five-year molar had started to break through, I assumed it was an abscessed tooth and took my son to our family dentist. We'd moved north to Worthington, Minnesota, only a few weeks before and still considered Storm Lake home. My parents also lived in the small town, just blocks from Craig's mom.

After examining Jason, our dentist explained that the molar was coming in crooked and referred us to an oral surgeon. We made an appointment for the following morning. Nothing Dr. Duethman said, nothing in his manner, suggested this was anything but a simple, routine dental problem. At the time my only concern was having to tell Adam and Tim, Jason's brothers, that our trip to Worlds of Fun would be delayed.

The oral surgeon tried unsuccessfully to aspirate the abscess. Peering at Jason's X rays, Dr. Synhorst said, "I'm going to have to extract the tooth under anesthesia. Bring Jason to the hospital tomorrow, and we'll take care of it." I winced, not at the word *hospital*, but at the realization that this inconvenience would deduct another day from our vacation.

As Craig and I brought Jason to the hospital emergency room in nearby Spencer, Iowa, that Thursday morning, I remarked, "You know, taking out his molar is going to cause his other teeth to move around. I bet he'll have to wear braces when he's older." That was the worst thing I could think of.

Anticipating an hour's wait, Craig got us a container of popcorn. We'd barely munched any—maybe fifteen minutes had passed—when the receptionist announced that Dr. Synhorst and his colleague, Dr. Jorgensen, wanted to see us. "That's too soon," I murmured worriedly. "Something's the matter."

A nurse showed us to a cramped consultation room. Then the two physicians walked in and took seats across from us. Dr. Synhorst is a small, fine-boned man, always impeccably dressed and very distinguished, whereas Dr. Jorgensen is more casual, resembling a tall, lean

Texan in cowboy boots and a wide-brimmed Stetson. Though they made a mismatched pair, both wore identically solemn expressions.

"What we found," Dr. Synhorst began, "was a *lymphoma.*" Lymphoma? The word didn't register, but I sensed this was not information he wanted to impart.

"Well, is he going to have to spend the night?" my husband asked. "Or can we give him antibiotics on the road, because we were planning to leave for Worlds of Fun tomorrow."

The two men glanced at each other as if telepathically drawing straws to decide who would speak next.

"What we found, Mr. Gaes," said Dr. Synhorst, "was a malignancy."

I gasped, *lymphoma* and *malignancy* suddenly intersecting in my mind. But Craig, certainly not anticipating a diagnosis of cancer—from an oral surgeon? for a six-year-old boy?—still didn't grasp its implications.

"It never even dawned on me that Jason might have cancer," he recalls. "The surgeon kept coming up with these big words. *Malignant. Lymphoma. So what?* I thought. *I brought my son here to have a tooth pulled. Let's go. We've got a vacation to get on to.*"

My husband repeated, "Is it going to require medication?" When the doctors wouldn't meet his gaze, he turned to me, baffled.

"Craig," I said in a trembling voice, "they're telling us Jason has cancer."

Interestingly neither doctor once used that word, perhaps mindful that to most people a verdict of cancer constituted a virtual death sentence. In talking to other parents whose children have or had the disease, I find this is still a common thread. Medical professionals will say *lymphoma,* they'll say *sarcoma,* but few will ever say *cancer.*

From the moment a child is diagnosed with cancer, parents are forced to make countless critical medical decisions. As we sat there dazed and distraught, Drs. Synhorst and Jorgensen quietly explained that because the small Spencer hospital did not specialize in treating pediatric cancer, we'd have to take Jason elsewhere. They reeled off a list of approved cancer programs in Iowa, Minnesota, and South Dakota.

Though it is located clear across the state from Worthington, the renowned Mayo Clinic in Rochester was the only medical center my husband or I considered. Throughout this book we will stress the importance of making informed decisions. Knowing little about cancer at the time, however, we had to rely on instinct. To us the Mayo represented Jason's best chance for survival.

"Rochester," I said numbly. "We'll take him to Rochester." The two doctors politely excused themselves and went off to call ahead on our behalf, leaving Craig and me to cry in each other's arms.

I don't remember how long we sat in that room, but eventually we asked to see Jason, who was in the recovery ward, still under anesthesia. At a pay phone across the hall Craig dialed my parents to relay the dreadful news.

"When Geralyn's mother came to the phone," he remembers, "I said, 'This is Craig.' Then I started to cry. She asked over and over, 'Craig! Craig! What's the matter?' But I couldn't talk. It was like I was paralyzed. Finally I handed the phone to Geralyn, and she told her mother. I just couldn't do it. I guess I wasn't the big macho man I'd always thought I was."

Back in recovery we waited for our son to wake up, Craig pacing the floor, me sitting with my head resting on Jason's chest. It seemed like an eternity, but after about an hour and a half he stirred. "Mom," he said groggily, "I have this funny bump in my stomach." Panicked, I pulled another doctor out of the hallway. To this day I don't even know his name.

The physician gently examined Jason's abdomen with his hands and discovered a golfball-size lump that he feared was also malignant. Now, when the oral surgeons told us about the tumor in the mouth, I tried to be optimistic. No matter how dire the prognosis, I don't think you ever lose hope. I thought to myself, *They've made wonderful strides in treating cancer. They have all these new medicines. Okay, we can deal with this.* But when the second growth was found, a chilling fear surged through my body. I was terrified that Jason was full of cancer, which, as we would learn the next day, wasn't far from the truth.

Just then a nurse poked her head in the room to say she'd made us an appointment at the Mayo Clinic early the following week.

"You call them right back and tell them we'll be there in three hours," I barked. In a blur Jason's intravenous tube was disconnected, Craig tenderly scooped him up in his arms, wrapped him in a blanket, and rushed out to our van.

My husband's entire family came with us: brothers Terry, Tom, and

Kirk; Tom's wife, Susan; Kirk's then fiancée, Tammy; and Craig's mother, who sat holding our ten-month-old daughter, Melissa. I laid down in back with Jason, stroking his face and bright blond hair. He was scared, having been told he'd wake up in a hospital room.

"Mom, where are we going?"

"To Rochester." We'd taken Jason to the Mayo before, for a minor migraine headache problem.

"Why?"

"Because, honey, what they found in your mouth is something called cancer."

Other than that it was an eerily quiet ride down Interstate 90. As Craig raced east through the night at eighty-five miles per hour, the word *death* flashed on and off in his mind like a roadside neon sign. "I felt sick to my stomach, thinking about all the things we wouldn't get to do together," he recalls. "There wouldn't be any playing football with Jason, no basketball, no walking on the football field with him on Father's Night at school, nothing like that. I wondered if we would ever get to do any of the things we used to."

My own feelings can best be expressed in a metaphor: like we were careening down the side of a mountain in a car with no brakes. I knew what awaited us at the bottom, and there was no way to stop it. Considering how rapidly the stomach tumor had grown, seeming to materialize overnight, I feared that with every passing minute death pulled Jason farther from us. By the time we pulled up at Saint Marys Hospital, our son's tumor had literally doubled in size.

Saint Marys, one of two hospitals affiliated with the Mayo Clinic, specializes in pediatric surgery. A tiny twenty-seven-bed hospital when opened in 1889, it is now one of the world's largest private nonprofit facilities, serving over thirty-four thousand Mayo Clinic patients annually. The main building is a magnificent brick structure topped by a brightly illumined cupola that guides you up Second Street Southwest like a beacon. Just catching sight of it is somehow reassuring.

The automatic doors to the emergency room parted, and we rushed inside, the blinding fluorescent lights stinging our eyes. So many people bustled about, you'd have thought it was one o'clock in the afternoon, not ten o'clock at night. A stocky woman physician with boyishly styled sandy hair hastened over.

"I'm the one that spoke to the oral surgeon in Spencer," she said.

"I've been waiting for you." Today a pediatric hematologist-oncologist at the University of Virginia Medical Center in Charlottesville, Karen Bringelsen was then a Mayo resident who happened to be on call that Thursday night. "Dr. Karen," as Jason still affectionately calls her, would become an extremely important person in our lives.

While we were in transit, she'd spoken to Dr. Synhorst, who remarked that he'd examined Jason only yesterday and that he appeared fine. "When he told me another lump had been discovered in the abdomen," she recalls, "bells rang in my head: *Burkitt's lymphoma.*" Burkitt's, rare in this country, is one of the fastest growing, most aggressive of human cancers.

Dr. Bringelsen led Jason into an examination room and quickly verified the earlier diagnosis of a tumor. "About the size of a grapefruit," she calculated. Confirming whether or not it was Burkitt's required sending a tissue sample, or *biopsy,* to the hospital *pathologist,* a doctor specializing in identifying diseases through microscopic study.

Biopsies are carried out through one of the following methods: a minute sample may be scraped, like a Pap smear. In a needle-aspiration biopsy a fine- or wide-needle instrument is used to suction out cells. In an incisional biopsy a slice of tissue is cut out. Both procedures require local anesthesia. Jason had undergone an excisional biopsy, performed in an operating room under general anesthesia. Drs. Synhorst and Jorgensen removed the entire growth as well as his crooked molar.

In our haste to get to Rochester, we'd apparently dashed out of the Spencer hospital before anyone had a chance to give us the biopsied tumor. So Dr. Bringelsen dispatched two state troopers back there to collect it, a six-hour roundtrip. The prospect of having to wait until morning for a firm diagnosis was upsetting, given Dr. Bringelsen's suspicion of Burkitt's.

Both Craig and I come from large, extremely close-knit families, and by this time the waiting area hummed with some two dozen anxious relatives. My brother Mike, a tall, broad-shouldered businessman with a terrific sense of humor, joined us in the examination room and tried to cheer up his nephew. Doctors had been buzzing in and out all night, drawing blood. Lying on a gurney, his arm aching from the needles, our six-year-old was not a happy camper.

"You know, Jake," Mike said, digging something out of his pocket, "when I was five years old and lost my tooth, I got about a buck for it.

Now, seeing as how you had an operation to take yours out, I think it must be worth about, say, fifty dollars.''

"What's that you're holding?" Dr. Bringelsen asked suddenly.

It was Jason's tooth! I was so frazzled that I didn't recall having taken the extracted molar with us after all. In a fog I must have handed it to my brother earlier that evening. Dr. Bringelsen practically snatched the tooth from Mike's fingers and rushed it to the pathology lab. Thirty minutes later she returned with a definitive verdict: Burkitt's lymphoma.

As it was now well past midnight, the doctor let us go until early morning, when we were to report to the Mayo Clinic for a battery of tests. All two dozen of us staggered out into the breezy night air to find rooms at a nearby motel. Craig and I were so exhausted, we collapsed wearily into bed and fell sound asleep.

Waking up around dawn, I felt a momentary reprieve. *Did that really happen yesterday? I hope not, because that was the worst nightmare I ever had.*

Then I glanced around the strange motel room, remembered where we were and why, and all the anxiety and depression came swooping back down. Anyone who's experienced a loved one's death or a similar misfortune knows the crushing physical sensation that seems to clamp your entire body. As I climbed out of bed, my bones felt heavy, yet hollow.

The Mayo Clinic, six blocks east of Saint Marys Hospital, is actually a sprawling campus of sixteen buildings and parking ramps connected by an underground subway. The majestic Plummer Building instantly attracts your eye, particularly at night, when its breathtaking carillon is bathed in golden light. Though imposing at first, the Mayo is designed on a very human scale, with conspicuously posted maps and clearly marked signs, keeping visitors' confusion to a minimum. By your second or third visit you can navigate the Byzantine complex with relative ease.

Our first stop was the Mayo Building's pediatric oncology wing, 12A, which would come to feel like a second home over the next few years. (*Oncology* is the study of cancer; *pediatrics,* the branch of medicine pertaining to babies' and children's medical care.) A nurse handed us appointment cards, and for the next five hours we whisked Jason from one test to another: more blood tests, ultrasound, chest X ray, bonemarrow aspiration, CAT scan.

All morning I drifted about in a daze. None of this felt real. But during the chest X ray the reality that our son might die truly set in. I was standing alone in the cubicle where I'd undressed Jason and helped him into his little examination gown. As I bent down to pick up his clothes, it struck me that one day these might be all we'd have left of him. First I erupted in tears. Then I started screaming. A kind nurse, hearing the commotion, walked in, closed the door behind her, and wrapped her arms around me.

Sometime that afternoon Dr. Bringelsen and Dr. Omer Burgert took Craig and me aside to outline the situation. Dr. Burgert, along with Dr. Gerald Gilchrist and Dr. Tony Smithson, was one of Jason's three primary pediatric hematologist-oncologists. (*Hematology* is the study of the blood and its related diseases.) The diagnostic tests, he said, revealed four Burkitt's lymphomas in addition to the one excised the day before: two on the right kidney, one behind the left eye, and one in the abdomen. Amazingly the latter growth now extended ten inches in diameter, distending our son's belly, while the tumor involving the optic nerve caused his eyes to suddenly cross.

Dr. Burgert went on to describe briefly Jason's treatment, set to begin immediately in Saint Marys Hospital. The Mayo is strictly an outpatient facility, with more than four thousand patients passing through daily; inpatients are sent to either Saint Marys or Rochester Methodist Hospital, both staffed exclusively by Mayo physicians.

Then the doctor asked if we had any questions. That's when I cleared my throat and asked, "Is Jason going to die?" bracing for his answer.

Sympathetically but candidly he replied, "If I am to be honest, I have to tell you . . . probably yes."

With that awful realization our family was plunged into an emotional maelstrom. I don't know if I can adequately convey how instantly and irrevocably the diagnosis of a child's cancer changes literally every aspect of your life. Jason was no longer a typical six-year-old but a child *with cancer*. And our once happy family was now one in deep turmoil.

A clock on the wall read 12:45 P.M. God, how I wanted to turn those hands back to when we were still an ordinary middle-class couple. I suppose you'd describe us as having traditional values, our lives revolving around family.

A month before Jason was stricken, Craig and I celebrated our tenth wedding anniversary. The two of us had been teenage sweethearts, meeting when he was nineteen and I, sixteen. My family had recently moved from tiny Kingsley, Iowa (population, one thousand), to Storm Lake, a friendly, picturesque community about an hour's drive from Sioux City. Craig had lived there all his life.

The two of us were family friends long before falling in love. His parents, Fred and Lea Gaes, lived a mile or so away and were among the first people my folks met in Storm Lake. Craig became best friends with my older brother, Kenny, with whom I performed in a musical group called My Sister and I. Virtually every weekend Craig accompanied us to dances and county fairs, helping us load and unload our equipment. As a result we got to know each other well.

I liked Craig; thought he was cute, too, with long dark hair, a leather jacket and a charming smile. But my sheltering mother wouldn't let me date yet. Whether or not that had anything to do with my husband-to-be's nickname, "Casanova," I don't know. Fortunately for me, Craig is tremendously patient and persistent. He plotted to win her over.

"I went out with Geralyn on a dare actually," says my husband. "A mutual friend of ours bet me that I couldn't get Geralyn Lanham to go out with me. 'Let's do it,' I said. Knowing that her mother was very protective, I started wining and dining her. I guess you could say I dated Geralyn's mom before I dated her! I'd buy Isabel candy on Valentine's Day, take her out for pizza, watch TV with her.

"Finally one night when the two of us were supposed to go to the movies, she said to Geralyn, 'Craig wants to take me to the show, but I'm really too tired. Would you like to go with him?' That's how we started dating."

By then I was already in love with Craig, and it was only a matter of months before he proposed. Both of us knew, though, that once again my parents presented the biggest hurdle. First he asked my father, John, for permission. "Whatever makes Geralyn happy," Dad said, "but you've got to talk to Mom." It took us a week to build up the courage to ask her. She gave us her blessing, for which we were grateful.

Craig and I wed on May 4, 1974, a few months shy of my nineteenth birthday, and moved into a small house in Storm Lake. Less than a year and a half later we had our first child, Adam, followed on October 12, 1977, by the fraternal twins, Jason and Tim, who weighed an ample eight and a half pounds each. Looking back, my husband and I sometimes wish we'd waited a little longer to start a family, so that we could have spent more time together alone. Viewing it another way, by the time our last child heads off to college, Craig and I will still be in our mid-forties.

Motherhood and touring proved incompatible, so I gave up the band with my brother. Craig, too, changed careers for much the same reason. Since high school graduation he'd hauled livestock cross-country for his father's trucking company, a three-generation business. Craig, first and foremost a family man, knew from his own childhood that long-distance trucking can turn fathers into virtual strangers. In a painful decision he calls "the hardest I ever had to make," he left his father to work more locally, first for my parents' mineral and premix company, then as a supervisor for a meat-packing plant in Storm Lake.

I can honestly say that our three sons have never given us any serious trouble. Adam is a jock and a natural leader, looked up to by his younger brothers. "Very tough," both agree. "The best in every kind of sport," adds Jason. Although Adam's school grades sometimes concern us, he's not as susceptible to peer pressure as other teenagers, a relief to any parent.

The twins are as thick as thieves and have been since infancy, when they used to sleep sucking on each other's toes. Naturally over the years they've acquired different interests and sets of friends, yet Jason and Tim still go everywhere together. Twins can be highly competitive and sensitive about establishing separate identities, but we've seen little evidence of that. In fact, when they were six or so, the boys would pick out identical outfits to wear to school.

Jason's and Tim's personalities, however, are as different as the color of their eyes, which are blue and brown. Tim, who likes basketball and wrestling, gets frustrated easily and is emotionally volatile, whereas Jason has always been accepting and even-tempered. Yet Tim is probably the most nurturing of the three boys. If I'm fixing supper and complain of having a headache, Tim is the one who goes and gets the aspirin. "Why don't you lie down, Mom," he'll say caringly. "We can have this tomorrow night. I'll just make us soup and sandwiches for tonight."

In Adam's eyes "Tim is very shy around people and doesn't talk much, while Jason is very forward and says what he thinks." How true.

Jason always seemed unusually expressive, freely asking questions and discussing his feelings. Even at age six he acted extremely mature, but in all other respects was a typical boy, crazy about G.I. Joe and Masters of the Universe dolls.

We thought our family of five was complete. But on my twenty-eighth birthday, August 9, 1983, along came Melissa, the first girl in my husband's family for several generations. As we waited for the doctors to perform a cesarean section, I whispered to Craig, "You really want a girl, don't you?"

"No, no," he assured me. "So long as it's healthy. My dad had four sons. Four sons would be great."

After the nurse wrapped Melissa in a pink blanket, though, my husband threw open the operating-room door and shouted, "I lied! I lied! I wanted a girl!" We were all thrilled with Missy.

One week later Craig took a supervisor's job at a new meat-packing plant about ninety minutes north of Storm Lake. Worthington, tucked in Minnesota's southwest corner, is a tranquil town, although not as quaint, perhaps, as our old community. The following May the kids and I joined Craig there, in a small one-story rented house near sparkling Okabena Lake.

It was a hectic but exciting time. You have to remember, neither my husband nor I had ever lived completely on our own before. As summer approached, I began searching for a permanent house. Basically we were working on our share of the American Dream: buying a home, saving for our children's college educations, looking optimistically toward the future. "Things were going really well for us," recalls Craig. "Everything was working out great."

Before the reality of Jason's cancer had even set in, my husband and I faced the grim task of breaking the news to him. Years ago parents and doctors shielded young patients from the truth. Or, I should say, deluded themselves by thinking they were protecting them, for kids are extraordinarily perceptive. To use a popular midwestern expression they know when you're blowin' smoke up their hind ends.

Eventually most learn the truth by eavesdropping on hushed conversations between parents and doctors or talking with other youngsters in the hospital. It's been found that children even as young as four can sense they are seriously ill just from reading their parents' worried expressions.

Dr. Gilchrist observes, "Most parents' first reaction is to hide the truth from their children. We still have the occasional mother or father who continues to resist our addressing the patient about the realities of the situation. Fortunately that's the exception, but it does create a lot of tension. Particularly with teenagers, you know damn well they understand what's going on. You can't hide your emotions from them."

According to one study, children whose parents leveled with them from the start fared better psychologically than those not told for a year or more or who uncovered the truth on their own. Is it any wonder? Kids kept in the dark ultimately grow more frightened than those who know. Many, especially young ones, fantasize scenarios more nightmarish than the reality.

These children are left feeling abandoned, betrayed, and lied to by adults they've trusted implicitly from birth. With the best of intentions their parents have condemned them to endure cancer therapy alone, with no one to confide in or to console them. Secrecy also sends a message that having cancer is cause for embarrassment, heaping feelings of shame onto an already overburdened child.

Further exacerbating matters, the strain of maintaining the silence may cause parents subconsciously to pull away from their sick children. It's an unfortunate situation all around. I can't imagine anything worse than a child dying and her parents forever berating themselves, believing they'd let her down.

Perhaps the most valuable advice any doctor gave us came from Dr. Bringelsen that afternoon in the Mayo Clinic. When I wondered aloud how I would tell our son what the doctors had discovered, she replied, "If you choose to deceive Jason, and he finds out, then he will constantly be afraid, because he won't be able to trust anything else you say."

Throughout Jason's treatment Craig and I were as honest with him as we knew how to be. If an upcoming test might prove upsetting or painful, we explained what he could expect and worked on ways to get through it as best as possible. That way, whenever we told him that another procedure was a piece of cake, he could believe us and relax.

Some parents ask a doctor to tell their child he has cancer. My personal feeling is that no physician, no matter how compassionate, can comfort a youngster the way his mother and father can, and therefore parents should make every effort to deliver the news themselves. Let me emphasize that this is strictly an opinion, based on *my* personality and *my* family's dynamics. There is no evidence that young cancer patients informed by a doctor are necessarily traumatized. You must do what feels right for you and your child.

However, it may be appropriate to enlist a physician if you feel you cannot get through this admittedly stressful moment without breaking down. Not that there's anything wrong with shedding a few tears. But to fall to pieces in front of a child, especially now, could convey a sense of hopelessness. It's scary for kids to see their parents, their protectors, lose control at any time. No matter who tells your child, be at his side. Hold his hand, comfort him, tell him you love him; do whatever you can to let him know he is not in this alone.

How soon should you tell a young patient? Most experts agree the proper time is within a day or two of diagnosis, when a plan of care has been established. I told Jason in detail about his disease and treatment that Friday, immediately after the doctors explained it to us. I didn't see any point in waiting, feeling strongly that he needed to know why all this was happening to him.

A helpful free booklet called "Talking with Your Child About Cancer," which contains general guidelines on how to broach the subject, is published by the federal government's main cancer research and information agency, the National Cancer Institute. You can order it by calling toll-free (800) 4-CANCER. (For the NCI's address and more information about its free reference materials, see Appendix B.) Or, since you'll want to discuss cancer with your child promptly, ask your doctor, nurse, or hospital social worker if they have a copy handy. Chances are they do.

If you need to rehearse what to say, do so until you feel prepared and at ease. But in reality, when having to relay such shattering news to a child, I don't think any parent is ever truly ready.

I began by saying, "Jason, the doctors found something in your body called cancer." Now, he didn't know what lymphoma was, didn't *care* to know, but he did have an idea what cancer was. The week before, we'd seen the movie *The Terry Fox Story*, the poignant, true story of a dying cancer patient's marathon run across Canada to raise money for medical research. Making the young man's trek all the more remarkable, he'd lost a leg to the disease.

Jason's eyes grew wide. "Are they gonna cut off my leg?" he asked, worried he'd no longer be able to play basketball with his brothers.

"No, Jason, because that's not where they found your cancer."

He thought for a moment. "Mom, am I gonna die?" His voice was startlingly calm.

This is what I told him: "Well, Jason, some people get a cold, and it gets very, very bad, and they die from it. It's called pneumonia. And some people get cancer, and it gets very, very bad, and they die from that. But not everyone who gets cancer dies, just as not everyone who gets a cold dies."

In explaining his treatment to him, I said, "The doctors did all these tests and found some more bumps inside you. We can't see them, but they can. And in order to get rid of these bumps, they have to give you some medicine that will 'melt' them and make them go away. Now, you're going to have to take the medicine for a long time, and sometimes it's going to make you sick." I believed that if Jason were going to survive this, he had to know what we were facing.

But I also wanted to convey optimism, especially with the tragic fate of Terry Fox still fresh in my son's impressionable mind. "The doctors at the Mayo Clinic," I said, "are the best in the whole world at treating kids with cancer. They do this all the time. And they have all sorts of new medicines and machines to help make you well." Kids need to hear that not everyone with cancer dies and that the outlook for patients gets brighter all the time.

Had Jason been older or younger, naturally I would have tailored the information to his age, maturity, and level of comprehension. How much do you tell them? Children will let you know. Kids up to two years old cannot perceive the concept of disease; their main fear is being separated from you. But preschoolers to first-graders can understand illness, if not cancer in particular.

Children in this age group sometimes believe they're being punished for having done something wrong. I can't say that Jason ever expressed this to us, but it's important to reassure a guilt-ridden child that he is not responsible for his illness. Another typical belief is that doctors will restore them to health in an instant, like some magical wizard on a Saturday-morning cartoon. Without needlessly alarming your young-ster, tell him these special medicines take time to do their job.

The older the child, the more detailed your description of cancer. Second- to sixth-graders process new concepts in relation to their own experiences. So when explaining cancer to them, put it in terms they can visualize. A common analogy, appropriate for today's videogame-obsessed generation, is to compare a cancer cell to a bad Pac Man who devours the hardworking cells that make the body function. Most kids in junior high through high school, able to comprehend abstract con-cepts, can absorb the rudiments of cancer that we introduce in Chapter Two.

Your child may react in a number of ways: with denial, optimism, and/or anger. Dr. Gilchrist, a Mayo Clinic pediatric hematologist-oncologist since 1971, claims that in his experience, "Kids really handle it a lot better than their parents." Jason accepted the news quietly, though inside, he later told us, he feared that he might die. Early the next morning, when his doctors congregated in his hospital room to discuss his treatment, our son refused to acknowledge them, stubbornly staring at the cartoons on television. It was as if he were determined to make this a normal Saturday morning, no matter what.

I decided that I would also tell Adam and Tim right away. The two boys had spent the last two nights at my friend Claudia's house in Storm Lake, unaware that their brother was seriously ill. All they knew was that Jason was "sick." Saturday morning my parents returned to Iowa and brought them to Rochester. In a hospital "Rap Room" I explained Jason's illness to them pretty much as I'd explained it to him.

Adam, then seven, cried openly. "Cancer? Isn't that what Terry Fox had?"

"Yes, it is, honey."

Wiping his eyes, he said, "Jason could die, couldn't he?"

"Well, there is that possibility." Once again, in telling children you must strike a delicate balance between realism and optimism. Here I repeated what I'd told Jason: that the doctors at the Mayo Clinic were some of the world's best, that not everybody dies from cancer, and that we were all going to do everything we could to make Jason well.

Notice I said *we*. It's essential to include your other children in this full-family crisis, as a way of alleviating feelings of helplessness. Trying to spare siblings the truth may produce the same detrimental effects that we examined in relation to young patients.

Six-year-old Tim countered Adam's healthy outpouring of emotion by barely reacting at all. He appeared stunned, as if someone had just slapped him. He didn't cry, he didn't ask questions, though I encouraged him to. He just sat there and stared at me. And when the conversation ended, he got up and walked away.

He's so little, I thought, *he probably doesn't realize what cancer is.* In retrospect I misread Tim. I think he did understand the gravity of his twin's cancer. He was in shock, a response that wouldn't wear off for a long time.

"At first," he remembers, "I thought cancer was like a flu; Jason would get a few pills, go home, and be okay in a couple of days. My mom told me it would be more than a couple of days; that it could be years, and that Jason might die.

"I thought to myself, *Jason, you'd better start pushing yourself so you can live, because I don't want you to die.*"

CHAPTER TWO

IDENTIFYING THE ENEMY: LEARNING ABOUT CANCER

Parents' Typical Reactions • Recommended
Resources • Cancer's Causes • Types of Cancer
• Diagnostic Tests

In the days after Jason's diagnosis Craig and I felt the gamut of emotions familiar to fathers and mothers of pediatric-cancer patients: denial, guilt, self-pity, fear, confusion, grief, hope, but especially rage. How could this happen to Jason, of all kids? He was so sweet, gentle, and innocent. It seemed the epitome of injustice.

Anger is a very natural, immediate reaction. Once the initial shock subsides, however, it can immobilize you. Because children's cancer strikes so suddenly, parents must make crucial decisions right away. You don't have time to ponder, Why my child? Why *any* child? Far more pressing are such questions as What can I do to best meet my child's needs? How do I locate the most comprehensive medical care? Where do I find up-to-date cancer information?

The why? question is less easily satisfied, often haunting parents even after their child's recovery. To this day I can't say that Craig and I have received a comforting answer. God's will? Plain old misfortune? As with other tragedies in life, perhaps it's best simply to accept that childhood cancer *just happens*.

My husband, boiling over with bitterness, had an extremely difficult time working through the anger stage. Only the year before, he'd lost his father, a wonderful, generous man, to a heart attack. Craig was as close to his dad as a son could be, stopping off for a beer every evening on his way home from work. "If I missed a day," he remembers, "my dad would call me up. 'Are you mad at me or somethin'?' I'd drive right over for that beer. The night before he collapsed and died was one of the few I didn't see him. I still think about that."

Fred Gaes's death at age fifty-nine devastated Craig. Now it appeared that someone else he loved dearly was about to be taken away. In a not uncommon reaction, he felt that he, as well as his son, was being unfairly punished.

At Saint Marys that first night my shaken mother suggested we all pray in the hospital chapel.

"You go ahead and pray," Craig replied stonily. "I'm all done praying."

My husband now says, "I was angry about God betraying me. At least I believed he'd betrayed me. I thought to myself, *I work hard, I take good care of my family, I go to church every Sunday. Meanwhile there are people who spend their nights in bars and go home and beat up their wives, and they've got four or five healthy kids. Why is this happening to me?*"

Eventually Craig's anger burned itself out. Overcoming the helplessness that envelops you following a cancer diagnosis, however, can take far longer. So much happens in such a short time, it's hard not to feel overwhelmed. One moment your life is pointing steadfastly in one direction, the next it's spinning wildly out of control. You see everything you've worked for disintegrating before your eyes, and you're powerless to stop it.

One way for Craig and me to regain control, even if it was merely an illusion of control, was to learn about Jason's disease. As far as we knew, no one in either of our families had ever had cancer, so the barrage of medical jargon the doctors threw at us might as well have been a foreign language. When Dr. Burgert said he wanted to start our son on *chemotherapy* right away—treating the tumors with highly potent drugs—I imagined some sort of futuristic cancer-curing machine. I'd heard of chemotherapy, of course, but had little idea what it was or how it worked.

Throughout Jason's illness I was astounded to meet parents who knew little or nothing about cancer or its treatment.

"What drug is your daughter on?"

"Um, gee, I can't remember." I suppose that for some people ignorance is bliss, exempting them, in their minds, from responsibility for their child's recovery. Success or failure can then be deposited solely on the medical team. Or God. Or fate.

As comfortable as that may seem, parents' ignorance jeopardizes their child's chances of survival. Many times I picked up practical advice from casual discussions with other mothers at the Mayo Clinic: trading tips on how to quell the nausea brought on by radiation and chemotherapy, or ways to make food more palatable. Also, if asked to consent in writing to a particular therapy for your youngster, certainly you want to make an educated decision.

Personally I'm a searcher, a seeker. I needed to know as much as I could about Burkitt's lymphoma, for my sake as well as for Jason's. Simply sizing up the enemy, I found, restored a degree of control. And feeling informed and that I was doing something, anything, for him, helped to offset that sense of helplessness.

LEARNING ABOUT CANCER

Metastasis. Blastoma. Immunotherapy. There are so many alien medical terms to absorb, but because they now have such vivid meaning in your life, you pick them up surprisingly quickly. (For unfamiliar terms, please make use of this book's glossary.) Craig and I found print information the most instructive; you're in such a state of shock early on that doctors' words often don't sink in.

The world of cancer and cancer therapy changes constantly. Therefore make sure that your reading material is current, no more than two or three years old. For that reason we recommend an excellent free series of clear, concise, and frequently updated handbooks on children's cancer published by the U.S. Department of Health and Human Services and available through the National Cancer Institute Office of Cancer Communications (800-4-CANCER); the American Cancer Society (800-ACS-2345); and the Leukemia Society of America (800-955-4LSA). Addresses for each are in the appendix, along with a list of suggested titles to request.

The National Cancer Institute's "Young People with Cancer: A

Handbook for Parents" is an excellent sixty-seven-page resource containing general information on the disease, methods of treatment and
how a child's cancer affects the entire family. Supplement it with booklets from the two NCI series on specific forms of cancer, "What You
Need to Know About . . ." and the more detailed "research reports."
Both list suggested additional readings.

The NCI also maintains the Physicians Data Query (PDQ), a vast
computer data base compiled from 150 medical centers in the United
States and twenty-two countries on the latest advances in cancer therapy. Housed in Bethesda, Maryland, it was developed to standardize
cancer treatment, so that a doctor in the smallest facility can instantly
access the same information on treatment options as a physician at a
major institution.

Only doctors can tap directly into the data base, but you can receive
the same statements by dialing (800) 4-CANCER. A trained staff person
will need to know your child's age, the type of cancer he has, its extent,
your hometown, and so on. From this he conducts a computer search,
then mails you a rather technical printout on treatment options. *Share
the "PDQ State-of-the-Art Cancer Treatment Information" with your youngster's
doctor.* Some parents worry that to investigate other therapies on their
own will offend the physician. As we assert in Chapter Three in the
section on dealing with the medical staff, if a doctor seems to resent or
belittle your active involvement in your child's health care, you may
want to consider changing physicians.

In addition to the aforementioned information services, your child's
doctors and the hospital social worker can recommend other reading
materials. Many are likely to have on hand several of the National
Cancer Institute, American Cancer Society, and Leukemia Society of
America booklets on cancer, as well as their own fact sheets and publi-
cations.

Naturally the public library is another source of cancer information.
Again, check the date of publication before reading. And while medical
journals such as the *New England Journal of Medicine* or the *Journal of the
American Medical Association* are certainly comprehensive, lay persons
may find them impenetrable and the language too arcane.

Telephone Information Lines

For instant answers to your questions, both the National Cancer Institute and the American Cancer Society administer toll-free information lines.

The NCI's confidential Cancer Information Service (800-4-CANCER) operates weekdays from 9:00 A.M. to 10:00 P.M. Eastern Standard Time.

For the American Cancer Society's information line, call (800) ACS-2345 Monday through Friday from 9:00 A.M. to 5:00 P.M.

Don't hesitate to use these services. The information specialists who answer your call will be patient and supportive and will have access to up-to-date PDQ information on cancer diagnosis and state-of-the-art therapy. They can also send you free print materials like the ones mentioned earlier. We will be referring you to these information lines throughout this book.

WHAT IS CANCER?

At some point during your child's fight against cancer you may encounter the well-meaning person who recounts the harrowing details of a friend's or relative's cancer. Your youngster is suffering from, say, Ewing's sarcoma; the patient being described, from adult lung cancer. Most people see no distinction between the two. They believe that cancer is cancer is cancer.

But cancer is not one disease, it's a group of over one hundred diseases that can arise anywhere on the body. Each form of cancer requires a specialized regimen of treatment, which it responds to or resists to varying degrees.

The Greek physician Hippocrates named the enigmatic disease some 2,400 years ago, but historians believe it plagued humankind long before that. Ancient Egyptian hieroglyphics and scrolls reveal that physicians of the day could differentiate between malignant tumors and benign ones. And while King Tutankhamen's mysterious death in the fourteenth century B.C. has been attributed to poison, some now say the young pharaoh's blackened stomach may have been the result of internal bleeding from cancer of the stomach or bowels.

Hippocrates' broad term can be divided into adult and pediatric cancers, which generally affect different organ systems. Kids rarely contract lung, colon, or breast cancers, the most frequent cancers among adults, while adults are largely immune to the childhood cancers Ewing's sarcoma, neuroblastoma, Wilms' tumor, retinoblastoma, and Burkitt's lymphoma.

"Cancer" is further categorized by gauging, or *staging* how extensively it has spread. Using a set of criteria unique to each cancer, a doctor assigns a patient's disease a stage, with stage I considered the most curable and stage IV the least. These classifications vary from cancer to cancer. For example not all stage II tumors are the same size. Likewise one patient's stage IV cancer may be more treatable than another's stage II cancer, simply because it's a different cancer or involves different body systems. We cannot stress often enough the importance of obtaining information specific to *your* child's cancer and to his particular circumstances.

The origin and nature of the disease, however, are constant no matter what the type. Simply stated, cancer occurs when one of the body's billions of microscopic cells develops abnormally. Whereas a healthy cell grows and divides systematically, a cancer cell multiplies rapidly and recklessly, over and over—$2 \times 2 = 4$; $4 \times 4 = 16$; $16 \times 16 = 256$, and so on—until the haywire cells begin crowding out, starving, and interfering with the functioning of the normal cells.

Eventually these rogue cancer cells produce excess tissue called *neoplasm*, also known as a *tumor*. A *benign*, or noncancerous, growth does not spread to other areas but stays *localized*. In most cases this condition is not life-threatening. The tumor is surgically removed, and the patient given a clean bill of health. The *malignant* tumor, however, is cancerous and can invade other tissues and organs, acting one of two ways:

- Invasively—the cancerous cells penetrate bordering healthy tissue yet stay as one mass.
- Metastically—a colony of malignant cells separates from the original mass and either moves directly to another part of the body or migrates through the bloodstream or the lymphatic system to distant parts. Then it grows and divides abnormally into new malignant tumors called *metastases*.

Malignant tumors may also be described as *in situ,* from the Latin for "in place." This is essentially a calm before the storm, a brief period before the cancerous cells attack healthy tissue. In-situ cancers are generally more treatable than invasive or metastatic tumors.

Tumors acquire the properties of the organ they affect. Of the five major classifications, three are solid: *carcinomas,* which form in the epithelial tissues that cover surfaces or line cavities; *sarcomas,* in the bones and soft tissue that connect, support, or surround other tissues and organs; and *lymphomas,* in the lymphatic system. *Myeloma* and *leukemia* are both cancers of the blood.

WHAT CAUSES CHILDHOOD CANCER?

Parents typically react to a diagnosis of pediatric cancer by blaming themselves, racking their brains for incriminating evidence. "We must have fed him wrong," they reason. "I sat too close to the color TV during my pregnancy." "We must have exposed him to harmful pesticides."

We know that adult cancers often result from controllable habits such as tobacco and alcohol use, excessive sun exposure, and a high-fat, low-fiber diet. However, thus far medical science is unable to conclude why young people develop the disease. Rest assured that nothing you did created this condition, and there was no way for you to have prevented it.

Genetics plays a part in some pediatric cancers, though we don't yet know how the disease or the propensity to develop it is transferred from parent to child. Forty percent of all retinoblastoma, a rare children's cancer of the eye, is believed to have been inherited through the genes. In some cases several family members may exhibit the malignancy. Another pattern suggesting heredity as a factor: the identical twin of a young leukemia patient has a 20-percent greater chance of acquiring the disease within two years. Siblings of children with brain tumors, sarcomas, and Hodgkin's disease, too, run a higher risk of those cancers than the general population. Despite these findings, the debate over whether or not some people are born genetically predisposed to cancer continues.

Two years after Jason was stricken, doctors diagnosed my elderly father with prostate cancer. Only then did I learn that two of his brothers had also had the disease and that two of his sisters and my grandmother had all died years before of other forms of cancer. I assumed this was due to heredity, but not necessarily. Cancer running in a family may be attributable more to its members sharing a similar life-style and diet than to genetics.

For instance, the people of Japan have a comparatively high rate of esophagus and stomach cancer. Yet Japanese who've relocated to Hawaii show a significantly lower incidence of stomach cancer, leading scientists to conclude that environmental causes have a significant effect on the population there. In our country environmental factors such as air and water pollution and pesticide and herbicide exposure are now believed to account for 80 percent of all cancers.

Thus far approximately thirty agents have been cited as triggering human cancer. Three of the most well-known are vinyl chloride, from the manufacturing of plastic; radon, a colorless, odorless natural gas that can seep from the ground into foundations and basements; and asbestos, a fibrous mineral long used in the manufacture of countless building materials.

In 1991 National Cancer Institute researchers confirmed a long-held theory that frying or barbecuing foods until they're charred can produce carcinogens far more harmful than the active ingredients in many federally banned pesticides. The NCI recommends that you cook all meats and fish at a temperature no higher than three hundred degrees and to braise, boil, poach, or microwave whenever possible.

High-voltage power lines and even household electrical appliances generate magnetic fields that, studies suggest, increase the chance of disease. Potential or suspected causes of cancer are omnipresent in the modern world, and sometimes it seems the only way to protect our kids is to dress them in a space suit and helmet.

Viruses have recently come under suspicion as another possible cause, although contrary to a long-standing misconception, cancer is *not* contagious. Scientists have associated viruses with rare forms of leukemia and lymphomas. Medical research is ever-evolving, though, and the theory that viral infections may contribute to cancer development remains unproven at this time.

TYPES OF PEDIATRIC CANCER

As Craig and I can attest, most parents of children with cancer are undoubtedly enough years removed from high school biology that explicit descriptions of the disease leave their heads swimming. Therefore we've tried to illuminate the major types of pediatric cancer as plainly as possible. You don't need to enroll in medical school to understand cancer, any more than you have to be a mechanic to drive a car. But it's essential to have a basic knowledge of the disease you and your child are striving to conquer.

In addition, this next section contains explanations of the tests used to diagnose and stage pediatric cancers. Many are not exclusive to one particular form. In order to avoid repetition, we describe these procedures in detail where they are *first* mentioned, on the following pages:

LYMPHOMAS

(Hodgkin's Disease, Non-Hodgkin's Lymphoblastic Lymphoma,
Non-Hodgkin's Nonlymphoblastic Lymphoma, Burkitt's Lymphoma,
Mycosis Fungoides, others)

The cancer Jason had, *lymphoma,* is classified into two types: *Hodgkin's disease* and rarer *non-Hodgkin's lymphomas,* a collective term for at least ten diseases, including Burkitt's. Hodgkin's disease usually afflicts young people ages fifteen to thirty-four, while non-Hodgkin's lymphomas strike children from five to fourteen.

Lymphomas affect the *lymphatic system,* which is part of the immune and circulatory systems. A network of vessels carries *lymph,* a yellowish fluid containing *lymphocytes,* into all the tissues of the body. Lymphocytes, one of three main types of mature white blood cells, are the body's soldiers against foreign substances—bacteria, viruses, fungi, pollen—known as *antigens.* These cells patrol the body, identifying and destroying antigens as well as dead and abnormal cells. When cancerous cells begin displacing normal lymphocytes, your child's ability to stave off infection and disease is compromised.

Hodgkin's disease and some non-Hodgkin's lymphomas originate in the *lymph nodes,* bean-shaped organs that, along with the spleen, act as sieves, filtering disease-causing agents out of the lymph as it flows through. These nodes are situated throughout the body, but are mainly clustered in the underarm, groin, neck, and abdomen.

Nodular lymphoma is characteristically *indolent,* spreading gradually. Most non-Hodgkin's lymphomas, however, form in *extranodal* sites— that is, outside the lymph nodes—for instance, in the spleen, bowel, gastrointestinal tract, liver, central nervous system, and bone marrow. These diseases spread more aggressively and diffusely, posing a greater danger.

Burkitt's lymphoma, rare in North America but common in tropical Africa, is one of the fastest-growing of all cancers. In African children it is usually discovered in the jaw, ovaries, and kidneys, and in North American kids, in the abdomen and neck. Jason, strangely enough, had tumors in both the jaw and the abdomen.

Symptoms of Lymphomas

- Painless swelling in the neck, armpit, or groin, caused by enlarged lymph glands
- Recurrent fever
- Night sweats
- Fatigue
- Weight loss
- Itchy skin
- Pain in abdomen, back, or legs
- Nausea or vomiting
- Enlarged abdomen
- Labored breathing
- Difficulty swallowing

Many of these symptoms, of course, indicate far less serious ailments, such as the common flu. One of the threats of Burkitt's and similarly aggressive cancers is that by the time a child exhibits signs—or by the time his parents suspect them to be possibly cancerous—the disease has already begun to spread, perhaps involving vital organs. Jason, for example, first complained of abdominal pain *after* his oral surgeons made the diagnosis of lymphoma. By then the tumor, comprised of literally billions of cancer cells, spanned an inch or two in diameter.

The National Cancer Institute recommends consulting your doctor if any of these symptoms persists for more than two weeks. Chillingly Dr. Bringelsen later told us that had we waited until the following week to bring our son to the Mayo Clinic, as originally planned, he probably would have died. We still thank God that Jason's uncle happened to notice the bump inside his mouth. Otherwise we wouldn't have seen signs of a jaw tumor until his cheeks began swelling, perhaps days later.

In the aftermath of diagnosis parents will sometimes fault themselves or their youngster's doctor for not recognizing the symptoms sooner. Almost always mothers and fathers torture themselves needlessly or accuse others unfairly. Because of the similarity to comparatively minor illnesses, the early detection of most childhood cancers can elude even medical professionals. And except in the case of rare, raging cancers such as Jason's, a few weeks' time one way or the other generally has little effect on the success of therapy.

Testing for and Staging Lymphomas

Kids suspected of having lymphoma will undergo *several but rarely all* of the following procedures:

- Biopsy
- Blood studies
- Body imaging: ultrasound studies, CAT scan, Magnetic Resonance Imaging, lymphangiography, gallium scan, nuclear scan
- Bone-marrow aspiration
- Laparotomy

Biopsy

The surest way to confirm suspicions of cancer is to biopsy tissue, in this case from an enlarged lymph node. By examining it under a microscope, a pathologist can identify the type of lymphoma. Hodgkin's disease, for example, reveals itself in a unique cell called the Reed-Sternberg cell. Once the disease is diagnosed, your oncologist will order a number of tests to stage its level. Staging is crucial, because each stage demands a specific type of treatment.

Blood Studies

Our first stop that Friday morning was the Mayo Building's hematology department, where a laboratory technician took blood from Jason's arm. Doctors then analyzed its components for abnormalities, such as a low white-blood-cell count or a drop in the protein *gamma globulin.*

The test takes no more than fifteen seconds but is rarely a child's favorite. Jason suggests covering frightened youngsters' eyes. "It doesn't hurt as much," he says, "when you can't see the needle." I'd either place my purse in front of his face or we'd concentrate on a wall clock and count off the seconds, a technique parents can work on with kids as young as two.

Blood may also be drawn from the fingertips, a simple procedure called a *finger stick.* In order to make the blood flow smoothly, the technician warms the finger by either rubbing it or having your child place his hand under his armpit. These quick pricks upset our son far more than a needle in the arm. He complained that afterward his bandaged finger felt sore, hurting whenever he picked up a crayon or fork. It didn't take him long to voice his preference, and after that blood was usually taken from his arm.

Ultrasound Studies

Next we went upstairs to the fourth-floor radiology department for a series of X rays. First a physician called a *radiologist* examined Jason's abdomen using *ultrasound.* If you've been pregnant in the last decade or so, chances are you've had *ultrasonography,* as it's also known, yourself.

The procedure is easy to bear, even for a six-year-old. Jason lay comfortably on an examining table while the doctor passed the transducer, a hand-held device resembling a microphone, over his body. Ultrasound bounces sound waves off internal organs and structures, forming video images (the *sonogram*) that the radiologist is specially trained to interpret.

As with the blood test, Craig and I were allowed to hold our son's hand. "Ultrasound was the only fun thing that happened to me that day," recalls Jason, who was fascinated by the on-screen images. The radiologist narrated what she saw—"These are your kidneys . . . and over here's your liver"—but was conspicuously mum about spotting abdominal and kidney tumors. This information Dr. Burgert would deliver in private after the last test was completed and the results assessed, as it should be. Resist the temptation to read anything into the technician's manner or facial expression; medical protocol forbids them from discussing with patients what they see.

CAT Scan

Doctors also took conventional X rays of Jason's chest and bones. Later in the morning we returned to radiology for yet more body imaging: computerized axial tomography, or *CAT scan* for short. It was not one of Jason's favorite tests, that's for sure. To sharpen the image, a contrast dye is sometimes either injected or dripped *intravenously* into the child's veins. Almost immediately Jason began vomiting—not only this first time but whenever he underwent CAT scans. The dye, he complained, made him feel nauseous and hot inside, a fairly common reaction. Yet other young patients report little discomfort.

After a brief wait for the dye to circulate through the body, your child lies down on a table that is then drawn into a sort of mechanical tunnel. A rotating beam X rays him from the sides, front, and back at set intervals, creating cross-sectional images on a monitor or a paper print-out. From these, doctors can determine both the size and the density of tumors.

Including setup time the entire procedure takes roughly forty minutes to one hour. Although CAT scans are painless, many patients feel claustrophobic or scared by the groaning and clanking of the machine's gears. Therefore some kids may be administered a short-acting anes-thetic a half hour beforehand.

Plus, no one, not even technicians, is permitted in the room during the scan, a practice that may be as traumatic for parents as for young-sters. Imagine the heartbreak of seeing your child—clearly afraid of the intimidating machine about to gobble him up—and being unable to comfort him. I remember peering at Jason through a glass partition and thinking how tiny and helpless he looked. From then on I sat with my son while technicians readied the scanner, reassuring him that I'd be right outside watching.

Other X Rays and Scans

Young lymphoma patients may require other X rays and scans. *Magnetic Resonance Imaging (MRI)*, a relatively new technique similar to a CAT scan, provides a more detailed cross-sectional image by way of a power-ful magnet linked to a computer. One of its advantages is that it does not expose children to radiation. As in a CAT scan, patients are slid into a chamber, but the MRI machine sheathes them completely, and that may frighten some children.

Lymphangiography, which entails injecting contrast dye into the foot, outlines the lymph nodes and vessels to reveal any abnormalities. The procedure lasts anywhere from several hours to a full day.

Children undergoing *radioisotope studies*, also called *nuclear scans*, either swallow or are injected with a harmless dose of radioactive material. Electronic devices then track its path. Observing how the substance disperses within the body tells doctors whether or not organs such as the kidneys, liver, and brain are functioning properly. Admittedly the term sounds ominous, and some parents fear that the ingested radionuclides will make their child glow in the dark. The fact is that these scans actually subject patients to less radiation than conventional X rays.

In a *gallium scan*, another type of nuclear scan, a radionuclide called gallium-67 is injected into a vein. As the dye travels slowly through the body, a journey that sometimes takes days, it highlights cancerous lymph nodes.

Bone-Marrow Aspiration

Of all the tests conducted that Friday in the Mayo Clinic, the *bone-marrow aspiration* frightened Jason the most. This procedure enables doctors to determine if cancer has invaded the *bone marrow*, the spongy material that fills the cavities of the long bones and produces and stores the majority of blood cells. Craig and I wish we'd known more about cancer tests so that we could have told our son what to expect—another reason parents need to educate themselves about the disease.

As we understood it, the aspiration was like a flu shot, only in the rear hip, leg bone, or the chest's sternum. Well, it wasn't. At all. The needle is long and hollow, for harvesting marrow. My husband refers to it drily as "the gun." The technician had Jason lie on his stomach, placed a pillow under his pelvis and numbed the area with a local anesthetic. Then she slid the needle into the iliac bone and began drawing out about a teaspoon of marrow for analysis.

"Jason shot forward on the table," Craig remembers, "and grabbed for me, damn near tearing the buttons off my shirt." He had to lean across our six-year-old and pin him down. Still wincing at the memory, Jason says of the test, "It was real quick, but I'd never felt so much pain in my life. I yelled so loudly, I think everyone on the whole floor heard me."

Laparotomy

If a diagnosis cannot be reached by some other method, abdominal exploratory surgery, or *laparotomy*, may be necessary. During this operation the liver is sometimes biopsied and the spleen removed and examined *(splenectomy)*. In girls, should the physician anticipate treating the cancer with radiation to the pelvic area, the ovaries may be elevated *(ovariopexy)* out of the X ray beam's path. Likewise, metal clips may be implanted to shield the left kidney.

By early afternoon, only five hours after we'd arrived at the Mayo Clinic, Jason's test results were analyzed and his disease staged. As we wrote earlier, stages are defined differently from one cancer to another.

Not only that, but three classification systems are presently used in the United States.

One doctor might express the severity of your child's tumor in a number from one through four. Another might stage it with numbers and the letters *TNM: T* representing the primary tumor; *N,* nodal involvement; and *M* denoting metastases. Numbers following each letter would indicate how many tumors, size, degree of invasion, and so forth. Yet another oncologist might characterize the disease as low grade or high grade. Confusing? You bet. Thankfully, a movement to standardize staging terminology is underway.

Because even subtypes of the major pediatric cancers may be staged differently, we've elected not to include the divisions for each. A number or a letter will probably have little meaning for you, so be sure to ask your child's oncologist to clarify where the tumor is located, its size, and so forth. However, to give you an example of how cancer is classified, the National Cancer Institute currently stages non-Hodgkin's lymphoma as follows:

Stage I: Disease is limited to a single lymph node or extranodal organ.

Stage II: Disease has spread to other lymph nodes; *or* two or more tumors are present or nodal areas are affected on one side of the diaphragm; *or* tumor has invaded the gastrointestinal tract.

Stage III: Tumors are present or lymph nodes are involved on both sides of the diaphragm; *or* primary tumor has infiltrated the thorax; *or* extensive disease discovered within the abdomen; *or* paraspinal or epidural tumors present. (A *paraspinal* tumor lies just outside the spinal canal, while an *epidural* malignancy is found inside the spinal canal, between the bony spine and the *dura* membrane covering the spinal cord. It may also appear between the brain and the skull.)

Stage IV: Disease has affected the bone marrow or central nervous system, regardless of other sites.

By any definition, the news on Jason was not encouraging. His disease was assessed as stage IV, the least curable class of Burkitt's lymphoma.

Suggested Reading About Lymphomas

From the National Cancer Institute (800-4-CANCER):

- "Everything You Need to Know About Hodgkin's Disease"
- "Everything You Need to Know About Non-Hodgkin's Lymphomas"
- "Research Report: Hodgkin's Disease and the Non-Hodgkin's Lymphomas"
- "PDQ State-of-the-Art Cancer Treatment Information/Childhood Hodgkin's Disease"
- "PDQ State-of-the-Art Cancer Treatment Information/Childhood Non-Hodgkin's Lymphoma"

LEUKEMIA

(Acute Lymphocytic Leukemia, Acute Nonlymphocytic Leukemia, Acute Myelocytic Leukemia, Smoldering Leukemia, Preleukemia, Acute Monomyelocytic Leukemia, Acute Monocytic Leukemia, Acute Erythrocytic Leukemia, Promyelocytic Leukemia, Chronic Lymphocytic Leukemia, Chronic Myelogenous Leukemia, Hairy-Cell Leukemia)

During the course of our son's treatment, Jason, Craig, and I met kids with every form of cancer, many of whom lived and some of whom died. A number suffered from leukemia. The most prevalent pediatric cancer, it annually kills about one thousand children under fifteen.

Leukemia applies to a group of cancers that originate in the blood-forming cells, mainly those in the bone marrow, but also in the spleen and lymph nodes. To understand this malignant disease, it helps to appreciate the functions of the blood and of the cells that comprise the bloodstream.

Briefly, the blood carries nutrition, oxygen, hormones, and other chemicals to all the body's cells, removes waste products, and fights infection in conjunction with the lymphatic system. It has three components: *erythrocytes,* red blood cells that transport oxygen; *leukocytes,* mature white blood cells, which regulate the immune response to bacteria; and *platelets,* disk-shaped cells that prevent hemorrhaging by forming clots.

Derived from the Greek, *leukemia* means "white blood," a literal description of its effect. Immature white cells called *blasts* oversaturate the bone marrow and displace the red blood cells, robbing the body of oxygen. They also block the production of platelets and mature white blood cells, causing bruising and profuse bleeding and leaving youngsters vulnerable to infection. These leukemic blasts then infiltrate the bloodstream and lymphatic system, sweeping toward vital organs such as the lungs, kidneys, liver, spleen, and central nervous system. Internal bleeding that would normally be stanched by the platelets can turn fatal, as can viruses ordinarily destroyed by healthy white blood cells.

Acute leukemias, which affect young, rapidly dividing cells, progress quickly. By far the most widespread among patients twenty-one and under is *acute lymphocytic leukemia* (ALL). Other acute leukemias are *acute nonlymphocytic leukemia* (ANLL), a type that includes *acute myelogenous leukemia* (AML) and the rare *monocytic leukemia, promyelocytic leukemia, erythroleukemia,* and *myelomonocytic leukemia. Chronic* leukemias, which spread gradually, impair more mature, slowly multiplying cells. Unusual in children, these include *chronic lymphocytic leukemia* (CLL), *chronic myelogenous leukemia* (CML), and *hairy-cell leukemia.*

Symptoms of Leukemia

Acute leukemias' symptoms tend to emerge suddenly, whereas the warning signs of chronic leukemias are more insidious and difficult to detect, mimicking those of other childhood diseases. Chronic myelogenous leukemia, for instance, is often discovered only during a routine physical exam. But generally parents should monitor children for:

• Fatigue, weakness, and irritability
• Pallor
• Tiny red dots on the skin
• Frequent, unexplained bruising
• Enlarged lymph nodes
• Persistent infections impervious to antibiotics

- Excessive bleeding from gums, nose, etc.
- Sudden weight loss
- Swollen liver or spleen, causing protruding abdomen
- Bone or joint pain
- Fever and flulike symptoms
- Appetite loss
- Night sweats

Testing for and Staging Leukemia

- Blood studies
- Cell-marker studies
- Chromosomal analysis
- Bone-marrow aspiration
- Lumbar puncture

Leukemia can be tentatively diagnosed through testing the blood for leukemic blasts as well as low levels of platelets, normal white cells, and *hemoglobin,* the red cells' iron-rich protein that transports oxygen throughout the body.

Cell-Marker Studies
For a positive diagnosis researchers must examine one or more specimens of bone marrow, obtained through a bone-marrow aspiration. By means of *cell-marker studies* they can identify the type(s) and development of leukemic cells involved, determining, for example, whether a child with acute lymphocytic leukemia has T-cell or B-cell ALL.

Chromosomal Analysis
Should doctors presume your child has chronic leukemia, they will likely order a *chromosomal analysis* of the biopsied bone marrow. *Chromosomes,* contained in each cell's nucleus, are the threadlike bodies that carry human genes. In this test a pathologist hunts for a defect called the Philadelphia chromosome, so named because of its discovery at that city's University of Pennsylvania School of Medicine.

Lumbar Puncture (Spinal Tap)

Kids diagnosed with acute leukemias must undergo a *lumbar puncture,* more popularly known as a *spinal tap.* Make that "unpopularly known," at least as far as Jason was concerned. Beginning his first night as an inpatient, he endured spinals every other chemotherapy treatment. These were done not only to test the central nervous system for traces of cancer but to inject anticancer drugs.

As in the bone-marrow aspiration a hollow needle is used to withdraw approximately one or two teaspoons of cerebrospinal fluid from between the lower-spine vertebrae. Though spinals aren't nearly as uncomfortable as the former procedure, our son dreaded them, often throwing up in the waiting room from sheer anxiety.

A doctor instructs the child to curl up in a fetal position on an examining table, nose touching knees, for the greater the back's curvature, the easier it is to insert the needle. Lying still and relaxing also helps, no easy task for a youngster. "It makes spinals go faster," says Jason, "but it's hard to do. Once I walked into the room, I always got nervous right away." The procedure takes between twenty and sixty minutes. Eventually we learned that closing his eyes, breathing deeply, and fantasizing about being anywhere but on that table helped to relieve the stress.

For his first spinal, performed late Friday afternoon, after he'd been admitted to Saint Marys Hospital, none of us knew what to expect. A nurse convinced my husband and me to wait outside, saying, "Sometimes it goes better if you're not in the room." I knew from the very center of my soul that Jason wanted his dad or mom with him. The moment I heard his piercing cries, I vowed never again to be dissuaded from what I know was right.

Finally the nurse came back out and said, "Maybe it would calm him down if one of you were in here." So I sat in front of our son and softly explained what had to be done. Afterward Jason complained of a throbbing headache, a common reaction, and couldn't walk. My husband had to carry him back to his room, keeping his body flat, which helps alleviate the headache. We certainly recommend that parents insist on being present for their child's first spinal tap.

Suggested Reading About Leukemia

From the Leukemia Society of America (800-955-4LSA, 212-573-8484):

• "Acute Lymphocytic Leukemia"
• "Chronic Myelogenous Leukemia"

From the National Cancer Institute (800-4-CANCER):

• "Research Report: Leukemia"
• "What You Need to Know About Childhood Leukemia"
• "PDQ State-of-the-Art Treatment Information/Childhood Acute Lymphocytic Leukemia"
• "PDQ State-of-the-Art Treatment Information/Childhood Acute Myelogenous Leukemia"

BRAIN AND SPINAL-CORD CANCERS

(Medulloblastoma, Cerebrellar Astrocytoma, Infratentorial Ependymoma, Brainstem Glioma, Cerebral Astrocytoma, Supratentorial Ependymoma, Craniopharyngioma, Intracranial Germ Cell Tumor, Pineal Parenchymal Tumors, Supratentorial Primitive Neuroectodermal Tumor, Optic Tract Glioma)

Brain and spinal-cord cancers are the second most common type, seen in all ages of young people but especially those five to ten.

The brain, of course, is the body's command center, regulating and coordinating all mental and physical faculties. Information received from the body's network of nerves is transmitted to the brain along a cable of nerve tissue, the spinal cord, housed in the bony spinal column. When cancer attacks the brain and spinal cord, or the *central nervous system,* it can interfere with vital functions, from eyesight to movement to thought processes.

Almost half of all brain tumors are benign, and those that are malignant seldom metastasize to other areas. But don't underestimate their danger, for brain and spinal-cord cancers tend to resist therapy and recur frequently.

Symptoms of Brain and Spinal-Cord Cancers

Pediatric brain tumors are difficult to diagnose. Unless a tumor lies near a major nerve center, it may lurk undetected for some time before the child displays any signs. And those warnings vary, since the regions of the brain have unique, specialized functions. However, persistent, painful headaches—the result of an expanding tumor exerting pressure against normal brain tissue—are symptomatic of all brain cancers. Should your youngster complain of severe headaches, alert a doctor immediately. Other symptoms to look for:

- Impaired senses of sight, hearing, smell, speech, or taste
- Nausea or vomiting
- Difficulty walking
- Seizures, blackouts
- Unusual fatigue
- Irritability and sudden behavioral problems

Symptoms of spinal-cord cancer include:

- Pain
- Loss of physical sensation
- Moderate to severe paralysis

Testing for and Staging Brain and Spinal-Cord Cancers

- Neurologic exam
- Electroencephalography
- Brain imaging: X rays, ultrasound studies, angiography, CAT scan, pneumoencephalography, nuclear scan
- Biopsy
- Spinal tap

Neurologic Exam

After first reviewing your child's symptoms, a physician specializing in diseases of the nervous system examines the eyes. Using an instrument called an *opthalmoscope,* the *neurologist* examines the retina and the optic nerve. The former is the eye membrane that receives the images "projected" by the lens, while the latter conducts impulses from the retina to the brain. A tumor infringing on the optic nerve will cause an apparent swelling condition known as papilledema. The doctor may also test for muscle function, reflexes, and nerve sensitivity, lightly pricking the skin.

Electroencephalography

Electroencephalography, EEG for short, is a painless test used to diagnose brain tumors. Between one to two dozen disk-shaped conductors called electrodes are affixed to your child's scalp with a special paste. Then a machine records the brain's electrical activity, with abnormal brain wave patterns suggesting a possible malignancy.

Brain Imaging

One or several brain-imaging techniques may be used on a youngster thought to have brain cancer, including a CAT scan, nuclear scan, ultrasound studies, and X rays, all previously covered in this chapter. While conducting the skull X ray, the radiologist checks for any abnormality of the skull bones as well as for minute deposits of calcium in the brain that might indicate a tumor.

Young patients may also undergo *angiography,* to study the arteries that transport blood to the brain. As in a lymphangiography, a contrast medium is injected into the bloodstream, though for this procedure anesthesia is administered beforehand. *Pneumoencephalography,* uncommon since the advent of the CAT scanner, is another kind of brain X ray, only instead of dye, air or gas is injected into the cerebrospinal fluid of the brain's ventricles.

Suggested Reading About Brain and Spinal-Cord Cancers

From the National Cancer Institute (800-4-CANCER):

- "What You Need to Know About Cancer of the Brain and Spinal Cord"
- "PDQ State-of-the-Art Cancer Treatment Information/Childhood Brain Tumor"

NEUROBLASTOMA

Neuroblastoma, a malignant cancer of the sympathetic nervous system, occurs only in children, usually those age five or younger. A baby may even be born with full-blown neuroblastoma. For some reason youngsters under one are twice as likely to survive the disease as older patients.

More than 50 percent of these tumors take root in the adrenal glands, located near the kidneys. However, neuroblastoma can also affect, in descending order of frequency, the eyes, chest, neck, and pelvis. Primary tumors in these sites are not as lethal as those in the abdomen.

Symptoms of Neuroblastoma

- Swelling in the abdomen, chest, or eye
- Listlessness, weakness
- Chronic diarrhea
- Pain in the abdomen or other areas
- Sudden weight loss

Testing for and Staging Neuroblastoma

- Intravenous pyelography (IVP)
- Blood studies
- Ultrasound studies
- Urinalysis, to test for traces of a secreted chemical substance called catecholamine in the child's urine, which can indicate neuroblastoma
- Biopsy

Intravenous Pyelography

Intravenous pyelography is an X-ray study of the kidneys and other abdominal organs, for which a contrast medium is injected into a vein and followed over a period up to twenty-four hours.

Suggested Reading About Neuroblastoma

From the National Cancer Institute (800-4-CANCER):

- "PDQ State-of-the-Art Cancer Treatment Information/Neuroblastoma"

WILMS' TUMOR

One of the most curable of childhood cancers, *Wilms' tumor* mainly strikes kids seven and younger. It is a cancer of the kidneys, the oval-shaped organs on either side of the spine that extract waste products from the bloodstream and produce urine for excreting them. They also secrete a hormone called erythropoietin, which modulates the development of red blood cells. A young child's kidney is about half the size of an adult's, two inches long by one inch wide, and weighs roughly four ounces.

Symptoms of Wilms' Tumor

- Slight swelling or hard lump in the abdomen
- Bloody urine, the most frequent visible sign
- Abdominal pain
- Pallor
- Appetite loss, weight reduction
- Low-grade fever
- Fatigue
- Vomiting
- Diarrhea

Testing for and Staging Wilms' Tumor

- Blood studies, to assess kidney and liver function
- Body imaging: intravenous pyelography, CAT scan, ultrasound studies, nephrotomography, selective renal arteriography, chest X ray
- Urinalysis, to detect blood in urine
- Bone-marrow aspiration

Doctors can often positively identify Wilms' tumor through blood studies and body imaging. An increased red-blood-cell count, for instance, indicates kidney malfunction. Usually intravenous pyelography is performed to disclose any suspicious changes in the shape of the kidneys, ureter, or surrounding lymph nodes. Sometimes more precise techniques are necessary, such as *nephrotomography*, which yields a three-dimensional X ray of the kidney, or *selective renal arteriography*. The latter produces an X ray of the kidneys' veins and arteries, for which a contrast medium is first injected into the bloodstream.

Should the diagnostic procedures reveal a Wilms' tumor, your child's doctor may additionally test the lungs, liver, bones, and brain, the most frequent sites of kidney-cancer migration.

Suggested Reading About Wilms' Tumor

From the National Cancer Institute (800-4-CANCER):

- "Research Report: Adult Kidney Cancer and Wilms' Tumor"
- "What You Need to Know About Kidney Cancer"
- "PDQ State-of-the-Art Treatment Information/Wilms' Tumor"

SOFT-TISSUE SARCOMAS

(Rhabdomyosarcoma, Leiomyosarcoma, Fibrosarcoma, Liposarcoma, Infantile Hemangiopericytoma, Synovial Sarcoma, Neurofibrosarcoma, Alveolar Soft Part Sarcoma)

Sarcoma, from the Greek word *sarkoma*, means *fleshy growth*. These solid-tumor sarcomas arise in the body's muscles, fat, blood vessels, nerves, and other connective or supporting tissues. By far the most frequent in children is *rhabdomyosarcoma*, which afflicts two- to six-year-olds, as well as teenagers between fourteen and eighteen. This fast-spreading cancer can appear anywhere in the body, but usually manifests in the muscles of the head, neck, genitourinary tract, trunk, arms, and legs.

Symptoms of Soft-Tissue Sarcomas

• Painless mass
• Swelling
• Bleeding

Compared with other types of pediatric cancer, soft-tissue sarcomas quickly divulge their presence, usually as noticeable lumps. Because they can strike so many different areas, warning signs vary considerably. A mass in the neck may cause difficulty swallowing or hoarseness, while frequent urination, urine retention, or bloody urine are characteristic of a genitourinary tumor.

Testing for and Staging
Soft-Tissue Sarcomas

• Biopsy
• Body imaging: X rays, tomography, gallium scan, intravenous pyelography, brain scan, bone scan, liver scan, lymphangiography
• Lumbar puncture
• Bone-marrow aspiration

Soft-tissue sarcomas are diagnosed through biopsy. Once the disease is confirmed, your child's physician will want to X-ray and scan for metastases to other parts of the body, using one or more of the techniques listed above and described earlier in this chapter. He may also order a lumbar puncture and/or a bone-marrow aspiration, to test the spinal fluid and the marrow for evidence of cancer.

Suggested Reading About
Soft-Tissue Sarcomas

From the National Cancer Institute (800-4-CANCER):

• "Research Report: Soft Tissue Sarcomas in Adults and Children"
• "PDQ State-of-the-Art Cancer Treatment Information/Childhood Rhabdomyosarcoma"

BONE CANCERS

(Osteogenic Sarcoma, Ewing's Sarcoma, Chondrosarcoma)

Bone tumors, the most fatal group of childhood cancers, occur in young people between ages ten and twenty-five, with a greater incidence among boys than girls. One reason these malignancies are so deadly is that they often speed through the veins to the lungs.

The two most prevalent kinds are *osteogenic sarcoma* and the rarer, faster-growing *Ewing's sarcoma*. Although sarcomas can develop in any of the body's 206 bones, osteogenic usually attacks the ends of the large bones in the upper arm (humerus) and the leg (femur and tibia), while Ewing's involves the midshafts. The latter type also differs in that it affects other bones, such as the ribs, pelvis, and thigh bone (femur). A third classification, *chondrosarcoma,* found even less frequently in youngsters, takes hold in the cushioning joint tissue, or *cartilage,* of the legs, hips, or ribs.

Sarcomas of the bone destroy normal bone cells, so that sometimes the limb must be amputated. One of Jason's best friends from the Mayo Clinic, a tall Nebraska teenager named Doug, had osteogenic sarcoma of the arm. His doctors replaced the diseased bone with an artificial implant made of a metal called titanium, the first time this technique had been applied on a youngster there. The doctors also surgically transferred, or *grafted,* a healthy bone from his hip to hold the rod in place. Today Doug is a college student with partial use of his arm.

Symptoms of Bone Cancers

• Firm swelling or pain in forearm or lower leg (osteogenic)
• Fever, chills, weakness (Ewing's)

Because bone cancers mostly strike active teenagers, their slow-progressing symptoms can mislead both patients and parents into attributing the pain and swelling to injury. Doctors may initially confuse the disease with a number of ailments, such as glandular deficiencies or infection. The fever, chills, and weakness signaling Ewing's sarcoma are even more deceptive.

Testing for and Staging Bone Cancers

- Blood studies
- Biopsy
- Body imaging: chest X ray, bone scan, CAT scan, Magnetic Resonance Imaging, lung tomography, liver scan, brain scan, angiography (to help plan surgery)

Bone Scan

Before this procedure a radioactive material is injected into your child's bloodstream. By observing how and where it accumulates, physicians can identify the location, size, and shape of bone abnormalities. Benign tumors appear smooth and round, whereas malignancies are oddly shaped, with irregular edges. To verify the diagnosis, the tumor is biopsied. If the pathologist finds sarcoma, expect your doctor to image other organs where bone cancers are known to metastasize, such as the lungs, liver, and brain.

Suggested Reading About Bone Cancers

From the National Cancer Institute (800-4-CANCER):

- "What You Need to Know About Cancers of the Bone"
- "PDQ State-of-the-Art Cancer Treatment Information/Osteosarcoma"
- "PDQ State-of-the-Art Cancer Treatment Information/Ewing's Sarcoma"

RETINOBLASTOMA

This rare cancer of the eye is found primarily in children under four. When *retinoblastoma* affects one eye, it is said to be *unilateral;* when it involves both eyes, as in one third of all cases, it is *bilateral.* For patients with bilateral retinoblastoma, an effort is made to save the vision in at least one eye. If the tumor is extremely advanced, the eye may have to be removed, but 95 percent of the time doctors can preserve a child's eyesight.

Symptoms of Retinoblastoma

- Enlarged pupil
- Constant squinting
- "Cat's eye" reflex
- Eye pain
- Eye reddening, swelling
- Impaired vision

By the time most parents recognize the symptoms of retinoblastoma, the tumor has usually affected half the retina and seeded cancerous cells to other parts of the eye. A mother we met at the Mayo Clinic told us how while rocking her newborn one morning she noticed an unusual white reflection, "a hole," from deep down in one eye. Still, she didn't give it much thought, casually mentioning the discovery to her pediatrician during a scheduled checkup. What she'd seen was the tumor itself. If the disease continues to grow undetected, eventually the child's eye may swell shut.

Testing for and Staging Retinoblastoma

- Eye exam
- Body imaging: X ray, CAT scan, bone scan
- Bone-marrow aspiration
- Lumbar puncture

Retinoblastoma patients are usually so young, physicians put them under general anesthesia before examining the interior of the eyes with an ophthalmoscope. Because the disease can metastasize to other, *extraocular,* sites, your child's doctor may call for a lumbar puncture and a bone-marrow aspiration in order to analyze the spinal fluid and bone marrow.

Suggested Reading About Retinoblastoma

From the National Cancer Institute (800-4-CANCER):

- "PDQ State-of-the-Art Cancer Treatment Information/Retinoblastoma"

ORAL CANCERS

Oral cancers, not generally seen in children, can form in any part of the mouth. They occur often in the lips, inner cheeks, gums, tongue, tonsils, floor of the mouth, and upper section of the throat, or pharynx.

The principal type of oral cancer, *squamous-cell carcinoma,* develops in the thin cells that line the oral cavity and the skin. *Basal-cell carcinoma* arises in the round basal cells in the skin's deepest layers, or *dermis,* while *melanoma* originates in the *melanocytes,* the cells that produce skin pigment.

Symptoms of Oral Cancers

The following warning signs are rarely painful:

- A mouth sore that won't heal and bleeds frequently
- Changes in tissue color
- A protruding growth, lump, or swelling in the cheek that your child can feel with her tongue
- White patches *(leukoplakia)* or red patches *(erythroplakia)* on the gums, tongue, or mouth lining
- Difficulty swallowing, chewing, or speaking
- Chronic sore throat, bleeding, tingling, numbness, burning

Testing for and Staging Oral Cancers

- Oral examination by a dentist or oral surgeon, including palpation of the lymph nodes in the neck
- Biopsy
- Imaging: dental, skull, and chest X rays; ultrasound studies; liver scan; bone scan; CAT scan; Magnetic Resonance Imaging; endoscopy

Usually an oral surgeon removes all or part of a questionable-looking lump, which a pathologist then biopsies. Only 7.5 percent of all oral cancers spread, but when they do, it's usually by way of the lymphatic system, metastasizing in the lungs, liver, and bones. Therefore your child's doctor may also want to conduct one or more of the above-mentioned imaging techniques.

Endoscopy

A flexible tubular instrument called an *endoscope* allows physicians to view inner body parts. Inserted through openings such as the mouth, the endoscope contains a bundle of light-carrying glass fibers and an attachable tweezerlike device for biopsying tissue. While the procedure is not painful, it is uncomfortable; therefore young patients may be sedated beforehand.

Suggested Reading About Oral Cancers

From the National Cancer Institute (800-4-CANCER):

- "Research Report: Oral Cancers"
- "What You Need to Know About Oral Cancers"
- "PDQ State-of-the-Art Treatment Information/Oral Cancers"

SKIN CANCERS

Though it does affect some young people, skin cancer is not a pediatric cancer per se, typically developing much later in life. We include it here because it is one cancer parents can help prevent by instilling in their children sensible attitudes toward sun exposure. The sun's ultraviolet rays are the chief cause of skin carcinomas.

The two most common carcinomas, slow-growing basal-cell and squamous-cell, rarely spread and are highly curable, but the more serious malignant melanoma can appear in other organs, including the eyes. Together these skin cancers account for one third of all adult cancers, more than any other. It is estimated that nearly half of all men and women to reach age sixty-five will suffer skin cancer, the seeds of which were probably sown during overexposure in childhood. That is when between 50 and 80 percent of all skin damage occurs. Malignant melanoma, for example, has been traced to just one or more incidents of blistering sunburns during childhood and adolescence.

According to the Skin Cancer Foundation, the disease usually strikes people with the following characteristics:

- Fair skin or freckles
- Blond, red, or light-brown hair
- Blue, green, or gray eyes
- A tendency to tan little or not at all, yet burn easily
- Many moles

However, don't be misled: Everyone is susceptible to skin cancer and should take the proper precautions. Keeping kids out of the sun or away from the beach, especially teenagers, is about as easy as keeping junk food out of their mouths. So the next best measure is to insist they use sunscreen, which absorbs or reflects most of the sun's harmful rays. The National Foundation for Cancer Research in Bethesda, Maryland, recommends that adults and children alike apply a lotion or cream of SPF (Sun Protection Factor) 15 for maximum protection. This is necessary even on overcast days, for 80 percent of the solar radiation penetrates cloud cover to injure the skin.

Other steps you can take include keeping children out of the sun between twelve and two P.M., Daylight Savings Time, when the sun's rays are most intense, or covering them with protective clothing, such as hats, long-sleeved shirts, and long pants. This is especially important for infants, who can suffer serious effects from sunburn.

Symptoms of Skin Cancers

The earlier the detection, the greater the chance of recovery. Should you notice any of the following warning signs, contact a doctor immediately:

- Discolored skin
- Changes in the size, color, shape, or thickness of preexisting moles.
- A new or old sore that won't heal
- A small, pale, waxy lump on the face, back, or chest, indicating basal-cell carcinoma
- Firm, irregularly shaped pink patches on the face, back, or chest, symptomatic of squamous-cell carcinoma
- A lump that bleeds or crusts
- A flat, scaly red spot

Testing for and Staging
Skin Cancers

- Examination by a *dermatologist,* a doctor who specializes in diagnosing and treating skin problems
- Biopsy
- X rays of the chest and liver, to check for spread

Suggested Reading About Skin Cancers

From the National Cancer Institute (800-4-CANCER):

- "Research Report: Nonmelanoma Skin Cancers"
- "What You Need to Know About Skin Cancer"
- "PDQ State-of-the-Art Cancer Treatment Information/Skin Cancer"
- "Research Report: Melanoma"
- "What You Need to Know About Melanoma"
- "PDQ State-of-the-Art Cancer Treatment Information/Melanoma"

From the Skin Cancer Foundation, 245 Fifth Avenue, Suite 2402, New York, NY 10016, (212) 725-5176:

- "For Every Child Under the Sun"

SURVIVING CHILDREN'S CANCER:
CAUSE FOR HOPE

The most salient fact to emerge from researching childhood cancer, you'll find, is that you have cause for hope, borne out by steadily improving survival rates. Just compare the National Cancer Institute's figures for selected pediatric cancers from 1963 to 1991, demonstrating the dramatic advances cancer researchers have made in the last three decades:

- Acute lymphocytic leukemia, from 4 percent to 73 percent
- Wilms' tumor, from 33 percent to 83 percent
- Brain and nervous-system cancers, from 35 percent to 59 percent

- Neuroblastoma, from 25 percent to 56 percent
- Bone cancers, from 20 percent to 54 percent
- Hodgkin's disease, from 52 percent to 85 percent
- Non-Hodgkin's lymphomas, from 18 percent to 68 percent

Much to my distress, a study I read in 1984 put the survival rate from advanced Burkitt's lymphoma at an ominous one in five. Incidently none of Jason's three primary doctors at the Mayo Clinic ever cited that figure, despite my prodding. Again and again "What are Jason's chances for recovery?" received the same even reply: "It depends on how he responds to treatment. Every child is different."

At the time, Craig and I wondered if Drs. Gilchrist, Smithson, and Burgert weren't evading the question. We now understand that what sounded like a pat answer was in fact proper and truthful. You will probably find that your youngster's oncologists, too, refrain from quoting statistics liberally, and with good reason. To begin with, studies don't necessarily present a complete picture. Of the patients who died from cancer, some may have been diagnosed late, or received a lesser quality of medical care, or failed to take medications as prescribed. These and many other significant factors aren't always reflected.

Dr. Burgert believes doctors "have to give people some kind of statistics," not only to help quantify the unquantifiable but to explain why a certain treatment is needed. "The key, though, is to explain to them the meaning of all these figures." He adds, "While we have an estimate from previous studies that a child has an approximate chance for recovery, new forms of treatment may improve the cure rate."

I think it's fair to say that relatively few parents are sophisticated statistical analysts, especially when they're distraught and desperately seeking answers. Understandably many focus only on the extreme outcomes—success equaling life; failure equaling death—and overlook the spectrum of variables that can influence a child's chances of recovery.

In Dr. Smithson's opinion, "Statistics have a way of becoming overpowering, whereas in an individual case you have hope." Perhaps some parents confronted with an 80-percent death rate would have given up. No question about it, those were formidable odds, but our family clung to the belief that Jason could be one of those one-in-five kids to beat Burkitt's. As the doctors patiently repeated, each case is different.

To illustrate, just three days after our son's cancer was discovered, another young Burkitt's patient entered Saint Marys Hospital. "Jill," as we'll call her, was an adorable four-year-old with silky blond hair, big blue eyes, and a charming disposition. She had one tumor; Jason had five. Both would receive the same drugs in the same dosages. Yet Jason lived, while, tragically, this beautiful little girl died a year and a half later. Given the circumstances the reverse outcome would have seemed more likely.

Disease defies logic and percentages, which is why you can't let statistics, no matter how discouraging, shake your faith. As Dr. Bringelsen tells parents, "It doesn't matter what happens to the other percentage of children. Whatever happens to your child is one hundred percent."

CHAPTER THREE

PARENTS AND PHYSICIANS IN PARTNERSHIP

Promoting Clear Communications • Treatment Protocols • Second Opinions • Selecting a Medical Facility

Apart from family ties, no other relationship is as important as the one you share with your child's health-care team. And it is a team, consisting of many skilled experts: pediatric hematologist-oncologists, radiation oncologists, surgical oncologists, nurse-practitioners, nurse's aides, X-ray and laboratory technicians, social workers, dieticians, and various diagnosticians, therapists, and medical specialists. Some you will see regularly, others perhaps but once for a specific test or procedure. During our son's cancer treatment we encountered dozens of faces, most of which passed anonymously in and out of our lives.

Then there were those that gradually came into focus, assuming names, familiar voices, and distinct personalities, beginning with Jason's primary physicians. For three years our lives and theirs were inextricably entwined, and no matter what our future paths, Drs. Burgert, Gilchrist, and Smithson hold a permanent place in our family's hearts. I think that would be true of anybody with whom you share such an intense, intimate experience. As Craig puts it, "We entrusted our child to them."

Forgive the generalization, but as most parents of recovered cancer patients will probably agree, the pediatric-oncology field attracts some exceptional men and women. I used to marvel at their ability to work in a stressful atmosphere where one out of every three young lives is lost, on the average, and grief follows euphoria follows grief in an endless cycle.

Dr. Gilchrist reflects, "We have our highs when kids respond to treatment and things are going well. Each time treatment fails, though, it's a real blow to every member of the team taking care of that child. It's very difficult to get off that roller coaster, and the truth is that no doctor is completely prepared to deal with it."

Physicians, like anyone else, respond differently to these emotional extremes. One may invest her feelings freely in patients and families, while another keeps his vaulted, appearing aloof and remote. This should not be interpreted as a lack of caring. There is no proper or improper approach, but you will likely find that you enjoy a more natural rapport with one physician than another. That's okay. It can take a while to adjust to each one's demeanor, especially with resident interns (and nurses) in training rotating every month or so.

Jason's oncology team was a perfect balance of contrasting personalities. Dr. Burgert, now retired after nearly forty years at the Mayo Clinic, is a tall, distinguished midwesterner. Though somewhat reserved, he was always very direct and a thoughtful, deliberate speaker. He went to great lengths to keep us informed, copying pertinent articles and cancer studies he felt we should see.

Dr. Gilchrist, the Mayo's director of pediatric hematology-oncology since 1984, is an avuncular-looking man with a resonant South African accent and a cheery disposition. I've never met a doctor more attuned to children. Now and then he'd breeze into the consultation room wearing a serious expression—and a huge rubber nose. As if nothing were out of the ordinary, he'd flip open his clipboard and begin discussing our son's condition. Jason used to go bonkers laughing.

Dr. Smithson fit comfortably between the other two. Though not as much of a kidder as Dr. Gilchrist, he was extremely personable and empathetic, the doctor most likely to squeeze your hand or offer a hug. He became "Tony" to us. A slender, handsome North Carolinan with penetrating eyes, Dr. Smithson came to the Mayo in 1974.

PARENTS, PATIENTS, PHYSICIANS: A PARTNERSHIP

There are three types of parent-physician relations, two of them detrimental for all concerned.

1. Some mothers and fathers unknowingly take an adversarial position, conspiring with the young patient against the doctors "who are doing all these bad things to you." Angry and frustrated over their child's illness, they blame the medical staff for setbacks beyond anyone's control. Ultimately this can undermine treatment as well as their youngster's confidence in her physicians. "We have to break up that 'us against them' attitude right away," says Dr. Smithson, "because that just does not work."

2. Other parents, intimidated by doctors, act overly submissive, like the Cowardly Lion cringing before the great and mighty Oz. They plaster a smile on their faces, believing that if they erect a sunny façade, they will be "rewarded" with better care for their kid. Conversely they don't ask questions for fear of "bothering" the physician, who, in their deepest unconscious fears, may then withhold treatment. This behavior robs the patient of an adult advocate who will question medical decisions and speak out when something seems wrong.

3. In the ideal relationship parents *work in partnership* with their youngster's medical staff. This takes effort and, above all, open, honest communication on both sides.

Ways to Promote Clear Communication

Ultimately doctors and other health-care professionals are people too. They cannot anticipate your every need and question, and it should go without saying that they cannot read your mind. While the responsibility of providing medical care rests with them, the job of establishing and maintaining good communications for the most part is yours.

• Begin by telling your child's doctors how much you wish to know about her condition and therapy and how you want to be informed about major developments. In person only? With your spouse present? A little bit at a time or everything at once? There is no right or wrong etiquette, only what best suits you. Any doctor worth his stethoscope will respect your decision and be grateful to learn your preferences.

• In consultations with your child's doctor, don't hesitate to ask questions, repeatedly if necessary, until you've absorbed the information thoroughly. Countless times I interrupted one of Jason's oncologists in mid-sentence. "Wait. Can you go back? I didn't understand what that meant." Sometimes I felt foolish, especially when he patiently reexplained it and I realized I *knew* that—it just didn't compute. But as Craig used to reassure me, "Geralyn, the only stupid question is the one you don't ask." The doctors at the Mayo Clinic, we both felt, always encouraged our questions.

Physicians realize many parents are self-conscious about appearing ignorant. And believe me, they've met with their share of reasonably intelligent adults whose retention suddenly plunges to elementary-school level out of fatigue, stress, and anxiety. Fielding the same questions, Dr. Smithson says simply, "is part of our job." Dr. Burgert's effective technique during discussions was to have us repeat information back to him, to make sure we truly understood everything.

• Because you never know how clear-headed you'll be from visit to visit, I recommend keeping a small notebook or journal in which to jot down questions as they occur to you. It's another phenomenon of parenting a child through pediatric cancer that whenever you speak with your youngster's physician, your burning question from the night before vanishes, only to return once you're driving home or the doctor has left for the day.

I'd suggest taking notes during consultations, but then you'd be too busy scribbling and not concentrating fully on the oncologist's words. A good idea is to have a less emotionally involved third party accompany you in the beginning stages, to act as your ears. Or tape-record your meetings, which Jason's doctors all agree is an acceptable practice. According to Dr. Burgert, "People make tape recordings of our discussions all the time."

• Some cautionary advice: Restrict your questions to those doctors who best know your child's medical history. Too many opinions, solicited or otherwise, create needless confusion and heartache. My husband will never forget a young Mayo intern who felt obligated to pull him off to the side that first day and implore him not to put Jason through the agony of treatment. Though unaware of the specifics of Jason's case, he brusquely stated, "Your son's going to die anyway."

"I nearly lost it," Craig recalls. "I thought, *Who the hell is this guy?* I'd heard this once already and didn't need to hear it again. I turned around and walked away, boiling."

What an unconscionably cruel thing to say! As it was, we were struggling to hold on to hope. My husband collared Dr. Bringelsen and complained. "Boy, she got hot," he remembers. "She said to me firmly, '*I* never told you Jason was going to die. I'm telling you that he's going to make it.'"

"She must have straightened out that intern," Craig adds, "because we never saw him again."

Dr. Smithson explains, "When parents come into a medical center, they are going to run into literally hundreds of people at all levels of training. All of them know their jobs, but they might not know a lot about pediatric cancer. The family has to realize this and not ask every person they meet about the medical prognosis. They need to identify who these people are and what their roles are."

He goes on to point out that because it was late June, the presumptuous intern might have been just beginning his three years' supervised training. The veteran residents had recently graduated to their own practices or into specialized areas of medicine.

This and other incidents, such as being discouraged from witnessing Jason's first spinal tap, taught Craig and me to assert ourselves. It certainly didn't come as second nature, for, like many people, I'd been raised never to challenge a doctor's authority. However, medical men and women are not omnipotent (though some of them might disagree), and parents must speak up should they feel the need to question a particular procedure's value or to object to unprofessional conduct.

From that day on if Jason's doctors said they were considering a certain test, I inquired, "What would happen if we didn't do that? What are our options?" I needed to know not only *what* would happen, but *why*. Never did I sense any resentment. Here are suggested questions to ask your child's physicians prior to tests:

• What is the purpose of this test?
• What can it tell us? What can't it tell us?

- Please explain the procedure from start to finish.
- Will it be conducted on an outpatient or inpatient basis, and why?
- Are there any health risks involved?
- Is the procedure uncomfortable or painful? If so, how can we help prepare our child beforehand?
- Can we anticipate any side effects?
- When will you get the results?

Asserting yourself doesn't mean antagonizing others unnecessarily. Speak your mind, but do so calmly. Like anyone else, doctors may react defensively to accusatory language or a harsh tone. Should a situation compel you to register dissatisfaction with your child's physicians, consider these ways of expressing yourself effectively:

- As your kid might say, "chill out," at least overnight. Discussions can turn combustible when one party's fuse is flickering. But don't wait so long that the urgency fades and you fail to pursue the issue. Similarly don't wait until you've accumulated a laundry list of questions, complaints, and grievances.
- Committing your thoughts to paper is always a good idea, particularly if you're easily intimidated. Construct a solid, logical case for your complaint, including suggested solutions to the problem.
- Relate your grievances in order of priority, and stick to one at a time.
- Rather than firing off vague charges, such as "I don't like Nurse Jones's attitude," offer concrete examples to substantiate your claims: "Nurse Jones didn't readjust our daughter's leaky intravenous line until almost two hours after I told her about it."
- Phrase your comments as statements, not indictments. Instead of, "You never return my phone calls," which is likely to prompt a defensive response, say, "*I feel* upset when I leave messages with your office and then don't hear from you for days."
- Persevere. Should the person seem to be skirting the issue, repeat how you feel.

Unless you've faced a medical crisis before, you're probably not sure just what parents should expect from their youngster's doctors. Based on a "Bill of Rights" promoted by the UCLA Cancer Center, physicians' obligations to parents and patients include the following:

- Detailed explanations of the patient's condition, available treatments, and other relevant information, if that is your wish
- Support, attention, patience, and satisfactory answers to questions
- Barring emergencies, spending a reasonable amount of time per visit
- Assistance in seeking other professional opinions, should you desire
- Keeping appointments
- Returning phone calls promptly, particularly those specified as urgent
- Making available the results of all tests
- Relating to you as one able person to another

Although patients under parental guardianship cannot legally consent to or refuse medical treatment, a child old enough to understand her predicament should be included in parent-physician conferences as often as reasonably possible. Once, one of Jason's doctors sat down with the three of us to discuss some tests results, the whole time directing his comments to Craig and me. Jason usually kept quiet during these talks yet listened with curiosity. After fidgeting in his chair for a while, our son suddenly piped up, "*I'm* the one that's sick. How come you're not telling *me* what's going on?"

I've seen this happen as well to ailing adults, such as my father, stricken with prostate cancer at age seventy. With Dad sitting right there, his physicians spoke to my mother and me about him as if he were invisible. My father rightfully complained. "I've been a successful businessman my entire life," he said. "Just because I get cancer, all of a sudden I'm an idiot who can't make a decision for himself?"

Ignoring patients or treating them like nonpersons, regardless of age, strips away their already diminished sense of personal power. Encourage your doctor to have a private relationship with your child. Our six-year-old loved it whenever Dr. Gilchrist kiddingly asked if he had any girlfriends (though Jason's response was always a predictable "Girls? Ugh!"). It made him feel good to be treated like a normal little boy. Kids deserve no less respect than adult patients.

Children's Hospital of Pittsburgh compiled for medical professionals the following dos and don'ts regarding young patients' dignity. Written on behalf of hospitalized kids everywhere, this sensible advice should be required reading for all children, parents, and health-care workers:

1. Since you know who we are, please tell us who you are and why you've come to see us.

2. Tell us difficult or bad news in private, not in public areas, especially not in play or waiting areas. If we cry or get upset, we'd rather do it without other people watching. We might also not want others to hear our news.

3. Take an interest in what we are doing and what we enjoy. We'd like to show you how special we are.

4. Don't examine us in public areas. This can embarrass us in front of friends and others. Do take us to a private area: our room or the exam/treatment room.

5. Our parents are important to us. Please understand that we may need them to be with us.

6. If we are busy working or playing, please give us a few minutes to finish before expecting us to go somewhere or do something else. This also helps us get ready for what will happen next. P.S.: Thanks.

Feeling neglected during consultations was the only complaint I ever heard Jason voice about his doctors. "All of them were really nice," he says. We couldn't figure out why at first he seemed to withdraw from Dr. Smithson, until we realized that for a long time Tony was the one who conducted the dreaded spinal taps. Jason associated him with the pain. Similarly parents may favor one doctor over another who in the past has been the bearer of distressing news.

Utilize the Social-Services Department

Sometimes faulty communication between parents and the medical staff blows relatively minor problems out of proportion. This is where the *pediatric-oncology social worker* figures into treatment, as an intermediary. Because of our excellent rapport with Jason's doctors, we had relatively little contact with the Mayo Clinic's social-services department.

However, things have changed greatly even since the mid-1980s, the medical establishment growing far more sensitive to the impact children's cancer has on families and the problems that can arise between them and their youngster's doctors. Accordingly hospitals now integrate the social worker into the treatment team more fully from the outset of therapy.

Dr. Gilchrist observes, "One reason social workers are such an important part of the team is that because they're not care givers in the medical sense, they can act as ombudsmen for the patient and family. There are many times when families are angry and upset with what their doctor or someone within the medical establishment is doing. They may have great difficulty verbalizing this, because we're also the people who they feel have 'the power of life and death' over them. So the social worker becomes a very important safety valve."

Today we doubtless would have seen quite a bit of Ginny Rissmiller, the caring young woman who joined the Mayo midway through Jason's treatment. "I think there's more of an understanding that we need to educate families about childhood cancer from the initial diagnosis," she explains. "We're there at the very first conference between the physician and the family to discuss the diagnosis, the prognosis, what the treatment plan involves, and the emotional impact this has on the child and family.

"We also ask all families to attend a pediatric-oncology education group that meets twice a week. It involves the entire paramedical staff—social workers, dietitians, Child Life specialists, chaplains, and nurses—and covers all the essential issues of pediatric cancer."

A pediatric social worker should have a master's degree or the equivalent, with additional training in coping with children and cancer. Consider him or her your personal advocate within the medical system, someone to help guide you through the unfamiliar terrain. This includes everything from building healthy doctor-patient-parent relations, to informing you about available financial assistance, to easing the young patient's return to school.

Changing Doctors

Sometimes no amount of discussion or outside mediation can rectify a lack of rapport. According to Dr. Gilchrist, "This is a problem many families have to face. After all, patients don't usually choose their oncologist. Even if they're sent to the Mayo Clinic to see one of us, if we happen not to be in, they're 'stuck' with the first person they encounter. I think it's fair to say that most people establish a very good relationship with that person," he emphasizes, "but we all have different personalities. In my opinion it's very reasonable for people to want to change doctors."

You are not wedded to your child's doctor. If at any time during treatment you feel the need to make a switch, do so. However, this is not a step to be taken lightly. Be honest with yourself: Are you genuinely dissatisfied with the level of care? Or by going to another physician are you secretly hoping to hear a more encouraging prognosis?

Again, if you've never been in this situation before, it's hard to know what constitutes unacceptable behavior. You may want to consider changing doctors if yours continually patronizes you and/or your child, dismisses your questions offhandedly, rushes through consultations, or seems unduly pessimistic about the chances for recovery. Often you can size up a physician by the deportment of her staff, who tend to reflect their employer's personality.

What if your child's doctor commits none of the above transgressions but his manner simply rubs you the wrong way or the lines of communication between you frequently cross? Personality clashes are no less inevitable in this situation than in any other. If you believe the gap between you is unbridgeable or could interfere with the quality of medical care, then by all means find another doctor. But keep this in mind: it's not essential that mothers and fathers adore their child's doctor, only that they have confidence in his ability and judgment.

Some parents tolerate unprofessional conduct rather than switch doctors because they fear that disrupting treatment in mid-course will jeopardize their child's health. This is simply not true. Patients change physicians, even institutions, all the time with no adverse consequences. Had Craig or I ever felt any reservations about Jason's medical care, we wouldn't have hesitated demanding a different doctor or taking him elsewhere. When fighting children's cancer, you have to do whatever you feel will best benefit your child. You don't get a second chance.

During the two years of Jason's cancer therapy we met with Drs. Gilchrist, Smithson, Burgert, and Bringelsen as a group just once: Saturday morning in our son's sixth-floor hospital room to discuss his *protocol*, the standardized treatment program for a particular type of cancer. Hospitals all over the country follow the same procedures so that results can be compared accurately.

Not too long ago surgery was the only effective cancer treatment. While today the National Cancer Institute credits radiation therapy with curing 25 percent of all recovered cancer patients, and chemotherapy, 15 percent, surgery is still the most common method, accounting for 60 percent of all cancer survivors.

A tumor that appears localized would be removed through what is called *specific* surgery, whereas a malignancy that has spread would require *radical* surgery, in which other affected tissues and organs are taken out as well. Surgery may also be used as a preventative measure, to remove a noncancerous growth or to ease complications brought on by the disease.

When initially told about Jason's five tumors, my immediate reaction was, *Cut them out. Just get them out of his body.* But except for the jaw tumor excised the day before, Jason's malignancies were inoperable. Many lymphatic tumors are described as *poorly differentiated.* That is, the cells' size and structure are irregular and their borders lack definition, making them difficult to excise cleanly without leaving behind malignant cells.

The doctors compared these abnormal growths' consistency to that of shaving cream, whereas *well-differentiated* solid tumors, such as a Wilms' kidney tumor, have a beefsteaklike texture and usually can be surgically controlled. Therefore they would attempt to shrink Jason's abdominal and kidney tumors with chemotherapy, which was begun that morning. A few days later they decided to treat the growth behind the left eye using cranial radiation. Both of these therapies are discussed in detail in Chapter Four.

Doctors will base your child's treatment protocol not only on her form of cancer, but on its stage and other variables. A young person with early Hodgkin's disease will usually be given radiation to the lymph nodes, yet one with advanced disease might receive a combination of four anticancer drugs. Please keep this in mind as you read the following chart, intended as a general outline of common treatment modalities for the basic pediatric cancer groups.

CHILDREN'S CANCER	THERAPEUTIC OPTIONS
Hodgkin's disease	Radiation and/or chemotherapy.
Non-Hodgkin's Lymphomas	Chemotherapy and/or radiation; in some instances local surgery.
Leukemia	Chemotherapy and/or radiation; in some instances bone-marrow transplant.
Brain and spinal-cord cancers	Surgery, sometimes followed by radiation or, increasingly, chemotherapy. Brainstem glioma may be treated by radiation alone.
Neuroblastoma	Surgery, often followed by radiation and/or chemotherapy. Disseminated neuroblastoma may be cured by chemotherapy, followed by surgery and/or radiation.
Wilms' tumor	Surgery followed by chemotherapy and/or radiation.
Soft-tissue sarcomas	Surgery followed by chemotherapy and/or radiation.
Bone sarcomas	Surgery followed by radiation and/or chemotherapy; sometimes radiation and chemotherapy. In some cases radiation is used instead of surgery.

CHILDREN'S CANCER	THERAPEUTIC OPTIONS
Retinoblastoma	Intraocular: one or more of the following—*cryotherapy,* freezing the tumor with liquid nitrogen; *photocoagulation,* heating and destroying the blood vessels that feed the tumor; external or implant radiation; surgery, usually to remove the eye. Extraocular (includes the tissues around the eyes or other parts of the body): radiation and chemotherapy.
Oral cancers	In most instances surgery, but increasingly, for early-stage disease, external or implant radiation. Chemotherapy is being tried in conjunction with surgery and/or radiation.
Nonmelanoma skin cancers	Most often surgery followed by *electrodesiccation:* killing remaining cancer cells and controlling bleeding through electrical current. Other methods include cryotherapy; radiation; and *topical chemotherapy:* applying anticancer cream or lotion to the affected area. Sometimes the tumor can be completely removed through biopsy alone.
Melanoma	Most often surgery; for advanced-stage patients, sometimes followed by chemotherapy. Ocular melanoma: usually surgery, often to remove the eye; also radiation or photocoagulation.

OBTAINING A SECOND OPINION

The American Medical Association (AMA) advises that before consenting to any medical treatment patients get a second opinion, something many insurance companies now cover. We did not, as Jason's diagnosis and protocol were established by a group of doctors. A second opinion? We probably received about a dozen in all.

There are a number of ways to go about this. Begin by asking your physician to recommend a pediatric oncologist. (If your youngster is already hospitalized, you might solicit a second opinion from a specialist on staff.) Though doctors should not take offense at such requests, regrettably some do. Should you meet with any resistance or resentment, a change of doctors may be in order.

Dr. Gilchrist of the Mayo Clinic notes, "We see a lot of patients who come here for a second opinion over the objections of their home physician. Often it sours the relationship. That is one of the most difficult situations.

"I'm always suspicious of any physician who reacts negatively," he continues. "My philosophy has always been, If I'm right, I'm delighted to have everyone else know about it, and if I'm wrong, I'd better find out fast." Even the renowned Mayo arranges for second opinions through other institutions when requested.

A *multidisciplinary* second opinion incorporates the views of several different specialists: medical, radiation, and surgical oncologists, augmented by yet others. Parents who want to hear all treatment options for their youngster can request a multidisciplinary second opinion at most major medical centers, where groups called tumor boards meet regularly to confer on individual cancer cases. Ask your physician to arrange for you to attend one of these symposia, at which he would submit the facts of your child's situation for discussion. In addition, some thirty cancer centers throughout the United States provide multidisciplinary second opinions, five of them at no cost. We've listed these for you in Appendix A.

Other ways to locate a pediatric oncologist in your area:

• Call the National Cancer Institute's Cancer Information Service at (800) 4-CANCER for free referrals. Its Physicians Data Query (PDQ) data base lists the names of more than fourteen thousand oncologists, including specialists.

• The American Society of Clinical Oncology (ASCO), whose membership consists of over eight thousand oncology professionals, also offers free referrals. It is located at 435 North Michigan Avenue, Suite 1717, Chicago, Illinois 60611, (312) 644-0828.

• Contact local medical societies, hospitals, or medical schools, or consult *The Directory of Medical Specialists*, available at many public libraries.

Two doctors' concurrence on diagnosis and protocol is considered sufficient to proceed with treatment. As with changing doctors in midcourse, parents who go off in search of yet another opinion may be subconsciously practicing denial, hoping unrealistically to hear a more favorable medical forecast. This not only subjects a sick child to unnecessary stress, it can hamper his chances of survival by delaying therapy.

CHOOSING A CANCER-TREATMENT CENTER

With treatment procedure set, you must next decide where to have it administered and by whom, for the medical center that identified and staged your child's disease may not necessarily have experience treating her form of pediatric cancer. This raises the chicken-and-egg question, which should you try to find first, an appropriate pediatric oncologist or a pediatric-oncology facility? Dr. Gilchrist recommends the latter, because, he says, "Virtually every pediatric oncologist in the country is affiliated with a major pediatric cancer center."

Craig and I never considered anywhere other than the Mayo, one of the twenty U.S. "comprehensive care centers" designated by the National Cancer Institute. Never did we regret our decision, despite its having been so strongly influenced by emotion and circumstance. While it's generally agreed that adults diagnosed with cancer have a window of two weeks in which to "shop" for physicians and facilities before starting therapy, children have no such luxury of time. What might my husband and I have done had we not lived within a reasonable distance of Rochester? What if there had been no clear-cut choice?

In selecting a cancer-treatment center, you must weigh several factors:

• Have its physicians treated many children with this particular form of cancer?

Since the advent of the National Cancer Institute's Physicians Data Query, all medical facilities are privy to the same state-of-the-art treatment information, reviewed and updated monthly by an esteemed panel of doctors and scientists. But in addition to knowledge, your child's physicians must have know-how.

Be sure that any facility you consider is staffed with a *pediatric* oncologist, which Dr. Gilchrist defines as "a physician who has expertise in treating the kinds of cancers peculiar to children *and* in dealing with children. Children," he emphasizes, "are not just small adults.

"Medical insurers don't always recognize this vital distinction," Dr. Gilchrist continues. "With the increasing pressures from a variety of different care givers, health-maintenance organizations, and third-party payers, there's this idea that, 'Hey, we have an oncologist in our group. Surely he can take care of a little kid.' " These otherwise capable physicians "know 'how' to treat the disease, they know what the 'recipe' is, but they really are not equipped to address the psychological needs and all the other needs of a growing child."

Health-maintenance organizations, conceived to provide comprehensive medical care for one all-encompassing premium, restrict their patients to HMO-authorized physicians and institutions. Sorry to say, families with this type of coverage have limited recourse should their HMO refuse to reimburse the services of a specialist outside its group.

If this happens to you, contact your state's department of insurance or department of health, both listed in the blue-pages section of your local white pages. According to our Minnesota Health Department, while its HMO Section has successfully intervened in getting HMOs to at least approve a onetime *consultation* with an outside physician, unless the family can prove medical necessity, seldom can it force HMOs to cover a *referral*. Still, complaints are considered case by case, making it worth your effort to report any disputed claims.

Recipients of Medicaid (public-assistance programs for those who can't afford private medical insurance) may find their ability to choose a physician restricted by its policies, as Medicaid limits them to vendors in their county. Furthermore, private-practice doctors are not required by law to accept Medicaid patients. Hospitals, however, are. Your alternative, then, is to bring your child to a county hospital with a pediatric oncologist on staff.

• The facility's oncology program should be approved by the American College of Surgeons.

The American College of Surgeons' Commission on Cancer has rated cancer programs across the country since 1956. For telephone referrals to approved programs in your area, contact the ACS's cancer department at 55 East Erie Street, Chicago, Illinois 60611, (312) 664-4050. Or request a free copy of its "Cancer Programs Approved" booklet, which is revised three times a year. The National Cancer Institute's Cancer Information Service (800-4-CANCER) can also refer you locally to Commission-approved programs.

Over 1,200 certified cancer programs operate nationwide, putting quality care within reach of most families. The majority are conducted in community hospitals, but also in freestanding cancer centers, teaching hospitals, and comprehensive cancer centers. These programs are not evenly scattered geographically, however. While California boasts 161, Montana has only one, bringing us to another consideration:

• The facility's location.

When your child is stricken with cancer, you would carry him to the ends of the earth for the best treatment. But today cancer therapy is conducted mainly on an outpatient basis for months, even years, making lengthy trips not only impractical but financially prohibitive. Beginning in August Jason had to go to the Mayo Clinic for chemotherapy every other week for a year and a half. Four in five patients there are treated as outpatients.

We lived one hundred eighty miles from Rochester, a manageable roundtrip day's drive. A distance much greater than that would have been almost impossible. Besides completely disrupting Jason's schooling and the family life we struggled to maintain, the travel and nights away from home would have been too stressful for him. Stress is potentially harmful to young people undergoing chemotherapy. It can depress white-cell counts already decimated by the toxic drugs, leaving patients open to infection.

Fortunately computers and information technologies have made it so that children can receive expert care near home. A practical solution for parents who want the benefits of a children's cancer center is to go there for diagnosis and stabilization, then find a local physician to continue the health care under the larger institution's supervision.

We did this to a limited extent by alternating our son's chemotherapy treatments between the Mayo and Worthington Regional Hospital, at Dr. Burgert's suggestion. Upon learning where we were from, he thought for a moment, then asked, "Isn't Benny Faul in Worthington?" Dr. Faul, it so happened, was our pediatrician.

"He's a wonderful doctor," Dr. Burgert said, adding that come the fall he would arrange for Jason's less powerful anticancer drugs to be administered there. Cutting our treks to Rochester by half certainly helped to ease the burden of our six-year-old's cancer, for every member of the family.

What if you feel strongly about including your hometown physician in treatment, but your pediatric oncologist won't cooperate? First, ask for his specific objections. If they seem vague and boil down to something on the order of, "That's just the way I work," find another oncologist.

Other Considerations When Selecting a Medical Facility

- Larger hospitals (of over five hundred beds) usually have more modern, technologically advanced equipment.
- Physicians affiliated with teaching hospitals are often more experienced with new treatment techniques and technology.
- Community hospitals in major cities tend to attract more medical students, an advantage over private facilities. They are also known to conform to higher medical standards than privately owned ones.

Hospitals, you'll find, have personalities. While Saint Marys was very flexible in its thinking, others can be exasperatingly rigid. It's amazing to me that some cancer centers still enforce the medieval policy that parents cannot stay overnight with their children. Come eight o'clock a security guard practically marches them to the elevator.

At Saint Marys the understanding staff bent the rules. For four nights I slept beside Jason's bed in a chair while my husband snoozed on the floor of the pediatric-oncology activity room, surrounded by a menagerie of stuffed animals. Though it was against regulations, a nurse discreetly left the door unlocked so that Craig could slip in and out. And I snuck into Jason's bathroom to shower, also a no-no, but the staff kindly looked the other way.

Worthington Hospital, on the other hand, forced me to test my newly developed assertiveness. One night a nurse came into Jason's room and curtly informed me I'd have to leave, since it was past visiting hours. With my young son pale and retching from chemotherapy, I was not about to go anywhere. Looking her in the eye, I said, "You can send security after me if you like, but I'm not leaving here." No one disturbed me again.

As of 1988, 98 percent of all medical facilities allowed for round-the-clock parental visitations, up from 76 percent in 1981. In the event that yours does not, ask your youngster's doctor to intervene or register a formal complaint with the administration. Some progressive facilities will install a cot in the child's room as well as provide other amenities. Whether or not a hospital has a kitchen area in which to microwave snacks may not seem like a big deal, but when you spend day after day there and tire of institutional cuisine, believe me, it looms large, as do visitors' showers, comfortable lounges, and adequate children's play areas.

On Tuesday, July 3, Jason's doctors gave him a week's reprieve before he was to return to the Mayo Clinic for his second dose of chemotherapy. Craig nearly sprinted out the door. I think he was as anxious to leave Saint Marys' pediatric-oncology floor as our little boy was.

"I hated that place," my husband admits. "Talk about being in a hallway of death." Young patients in various stages of treatment occupied the rooms. Some had lost their hair; others an arm or a leg. Still others were confined to bed, wasting away. Out of respect for their privacy—and, frankly, not prepared to confront the cruel truth of cancer—you averted your eyes when passing by those doorways. But you occasionally did glimpse a mother or father sitting rigidly by their dying child's bed, face taut with anguish, and you shuddered.

Having been through so much in five days, we were all just so relieved to be going home, even if only temporarily. And to see Jason up with his clothes on, playing in the back of the van with his G.I. Joes again . . . Well, it was a surprisingly joyful time. Tim and Adam, who'd been restricted to abbreviated hospital visits, were excited to have their brother back.

At home I immersed myself in doing the laundry, packing our clothes for the return trip to Rochester, cooking and freezing meals for Craig to eat while we were gone. It was a virtual repeat of the week before, when we'd been preparing to go on vacation, though I was too distracted to appreciate the irony. Everything seemed so deceptively *normal.*

A Fourth of July picnic jolted me back to the grim reality. Craig's company threw this big bash in Centennial Park, down the street from us. While Jason scooted around, giggling and playing with the other kids, seemingly oblivious that he had cancer, I listened to a litany of expressions of sympathy:

"Sorry about Jason."

"We heard about Jason."

"Bill told me about Jason."

And then these mothers and fathers hurried back to their own healthy youngsters. I'm not blaming them, mind you; we were new in town, and as often happens in times of tragedy, no one really knew what to say.

As I wandered among the crowd, surrounded by laughter and gaiety, this terrible, angry feeling welled up inside of me. I just wanted to scream, "How can you all be laughing? Don't you know what's happening?" Our family's world had just been blown apart like a firecracker, yet it seemed to elicit only an awkward "Gee, we're sorry." Neither before that moment nor since, have I ever felt more alone.

CHAPTER FOUR

RADIATION AND CHEMOTHERAPY

How They Are Used • Clinical Trials • Radiation and Chemotherapy Sessions

Sunday rolled around quicker than we would have liked yet not quickly enough. Though the five days at home were a godsend, Craig and I were anxious for Jason to undergo his second round of chemotherapy and to begin a solid month of intensive radiation, which his physicians had decided over the holiday would be necessary for dissolving the tumor behind his left eye.

Time was of the essence, we both knew, and the coming month critical to our son's survival. As we loaded luggage for the cross-state trip, we shared the same thought: this wasn't going to be easy for anyone, but the sooner we got on with it the better.

Compared with the previous week's panicked mad dash to Rochester, this drive took on the quality of a crusade. *We're going to the Mayo Clinic to make Jason well.* The pervasive feeling, I'd say, was one of determination and cautious optimism. My mother and the three boys joined me in the van, while Craig followed us in the family car with Melissa. Needed back at work Tuesday morning, Craig could stay only through the first day of Jason's radiation.

RADIATION

Radiation therapy beams high-energy X rays directly at cancerous cells, damaging or destroying them so that they cannot mature or divide, and, when effective, whittling down the tumor with each treatment. The bloodstream carries off these dead cells, which the body then excretes naturally.

Roughly half of all young cancer patients receive radiation. Pediatric cancers that generally respond well to it are said to be *radiosensitive.* These include early-stage Ewing's sarcoma, oral cancers, skin cancers, medulloblastoma, optic-nerve tumors, testicular cancer, retinoblastoma, and, in advanced stages, Wilms' tumor, neuroblastoma, and lymph-system malignancies like Jason's.

Radiation has been used in cancer treatment since around the turn of the century, though for decades its drawbacks nearly outweighed its benefits. Little was known then about the health risks of overexposure to X rays. This, coupled with primitive equipment, led to patients' receiving excessive doses that damaged healthy cells and organs as well as cancerous ones.

Since the 1950s several innovations have radically enhanced radiation's effectiveness. Highly powerful *megavolt* radiation from a number of sophisticated new machines deeply penetrates even the body's densest tissues. And the vivid computerized pictures produced by CAT scans and Magnetic Resonance Imaging allow specially trained *radiotherapists* to pinpoint the tumor's location and target the beams more precisely, preserving vital organs. Inevitably a number of healthy cells still get zapped, but these recover faster than cancer cells. That is why radiation is delivered in small, exact dosages over a period of weeks, so that inadvertently damaged normal cells have a chance to renew themselves.

In calculating the appropriate number of *rads* (short for *radiation absorbed dose*), doctors consider your youngster's age, sex, and overall health; the site and mass of the tumor; its rate of development and responsiveness to radiation; any surrounding tissues that may be affected; the extent of possible side effects; and whether or not the patient will receive chemotherapy simultaneously, like Jason. The dose also depends on how the radiotherapist intends to utilize radiation therapy:

- As *adjuvant* treatment, in conjunction with surgery and/or chemotherapy. It may be given to reduce tumors to a removable size prior to surgery, or to curtail the growth of stray cancer cells following surgery.
- As *palliative* treatment; not as a cure, but to shrink malignancies that may be causing pain or impeding bodily functions by intruding on nerves, passageways, or organs.
- As *curative,* primary treatment, to cure the disease or prolong survival.

When applicable, radiation offers advantages over surgery. Pediatric cancers that once could be stemmed only by operations to amputate a limb, remove an eye, or otherwise disfigure are now often treatable with no mutilation. Sometimes radiation is the only way to manage a local or regional cancer that's deeply embedded or in an organ that can't be reached without destroying adjacent tissue, as in the case of certain brain tumors.

A Radiation Therapy Session

Every weekday for five weeks our son received radiation to the skull. Once Jason got through his first few sessions, the treatments were a breeze. "It's easy," our seasoned veteran now tells other kids. "All you have to do is just lie there." Including setup time radiation takes between ten and twenty minutes.

That's if the day has gone according to schedule, which it frequently does not. Sometimes you'll arrive at the waiting area to find that the machine is down temporarily or that one patient's tardiness or another's emergency has created a daylong gridlock. It goes without saying that you should be on time to all appointments.

Expect to spend a good several hours your initial visit so that the staff can acquaint your youngster with the equipment and the procedure. At the Mayo Clinic's radiation-oncology department, says Dr. Paula Schomberg, "We let the kids ride up and down on the machine, to make sure there's no pressure. They're given plenty of time to get comfortable."

Besides determining the proper dose, the radiotherapy team must contour the radiation's dimensions, or *field,* to spare healthy areas. On a device called a *simulator,* a technician traces from your child's X rays the structures to be protected, at the same time cutting out a Styrofoam pattern. A lead alloy is poured into this mold and allowed to cool, forming a customized block that fits into the head of the machine and shapes the beam.

Other individualized molds, made of reusable plastic, plaster, metal, or other materials, are often cast to keep young patients immobile during the treatment. Our son wore a face mask that had ports through which the beams were aimed. Children under three and a half, or those who absolutely cannot lie still, are either sedated or given a short-acting general anesthetic.

So that the patient can be aligned correctly each time, a nurse or technician marks the target area with a colored dye, ink, or felt-tip pen. Jason's head bore four bright red *X*'s that designated the angles from which to radiate his tumor. Although supposedly indelible, they can come off if scrubbed. When washing the area, do so gently with a mild soap, then pat dry. To keep my son's head from getting wet during showers, I used to wrap a towel around it turban-style. Nowadays a clear adhesive tape is often placed over each marking, making it easier to care for. Should one fade, however, *never* try reapplying it yourself.

Wearing the *X*'s didn't faze our six-year-old in the least. However, adolescents, more self-conscious about their appearance, sometimes find these temporary "tattoos" upsetting, visible reminders of a serious illness. There is little mothers and fathers can say to cheer teens except to assure them that the spots will gradually disappear or be removed once radiation is completed.

In contrast to even just a few years ago today's medical centers are far more sensitive to patients' and parents' anxiety. Back when Jason underwent radiation therapy, parents weren't permitted beyond the waiting area. Now they are invited to sit in the brightly lit control room, talking back and forth with their child over a two-way intercom and watching her on a TV monitor. All around them computer terminals light up with the young patient's history, prescription, and other essential information that in 1984 was still recorded by hand.

As with any X ray you will be allowed in the radiation room only during setup. Your youngster lies on a mechanical table under the apparatus, which rotates 360 degrees to treat from any angle. I can best describe it as resembling a huge futuristic camera. Typically one of two types is used. X-ray machines, such as *linear accelerators* and *betatrons*, produce radioactivity electromagnetically. *Cobalt* machines, on the other hand, safely house a permanently radioactive metallic element (cobalt) and focus beams through a shutter.

The imposing equipment grunts and whirrs as it moves into position, which can be scary for some kids, as can the isolation. But the treatment is painless. Within a day or two Jason didn't even have to be coaxed into the room, sauntering right in on his own. Until your child gets used to the procedure, however, you'll want to reassure him over the intercom that you're right outside.

Bracytherapy

This method of radiation, rarely used on youngsters, involves surgically implanting or injecting a radioactive material near the tumor for up to fourteen days, then removing it. Unlike patients exposed to external radiation (which, contrary to popular misconception, does not render them radioactive), those with implants do in fact emit some radiation temporarily. In another form of internal radiation the material is left in the body permanently, soon becoming inert and thus harmless.

CHEMOTHERAPY

The following Monday Jason received his second chemotherapy, the literal meaning of which is chemical treatment. Generally the purpose of radiation is to impair or kill malignant cells locally or regionally. But chemotherapy usually fights cancer throughout the entire body, or *systemically*, by way of the bloodstream. Its mission is to pursue and destroy undetectable vagrant cells so that they don't multiply and form new tumors.

Like radiation these drugs don't distinguish between good and bad cells, damaging rapidly dividing normal cells as well as malignant ones. Therefore chemotherapy is dispensed in series called *courses*, with time off in between for healthy cells to recover. The first, and most intensive, course, *induction*, lasts weeks or months and is intended to wipe out as many abnormal cells as possible. Because the drugs' efficacy eventually diminishes, with the second stage, *consolidation*, oncologists often prescribe a new drug or combination of drugs to eradicate those resistant cells. *Maintenance,* the final and mildest phase, is for obliterating any remaining cells over a period of months or even years.

Chemotherapy is employed:

* In conjunction with radiation.
* To reduce tumor size prior to surgery or to destroy residual cells afterward.
* As a palliative measure for relieving pain.
* To impede or cure certain pediatric cancers, particularly leukemia and lymphomas. The medication doesn't need to eradicate every abnormal cell to be effective. Once the level drops within a certain range, the body's natural immune system can dispose of stragglers.

Widespread use of chemotherapy is a relatively recent phenomenon. It gained acceptance within the medical community after World War II, yet history shows that physicians tried to dissolve tumors with plant extracts over two thousand years ago. To date over 250,000 drugs have been studied for their chemotherapeutic potential, but only fifty or so have been deemed safe enough to give to patients—a 5,000:1 ratio.

For a long time it was a popular misconception that doctors used drug treatments only as a last resort. Today the Mayo's Dr. Smithson says, "People have accepted the idea that chemotherapy is part of the cure. This reflects the facts." Indeed. Each year chemotherapy saves some fifty thousand patients whom surgery and/or radiation alone cannot cure.

Clinical Trials

At our conference in Jason's hospital room the previous week, his physicians had explained that because different drugs affect cancer cells differently, they were prescribing a combination chemotherapy of four standard medications for treating Burkitt's lymphoma: cyclophosphamide, vincristine, methotrexate, and prednisone.

Cyclophosphamide is one of a group of anticancer drugs called *alkylating agents.* These interact chemically with cancer cells at all stages of development, preventing them from multiplying. Vincristine, a *mitotic inhibitor,* blocks malignant cells from splitting and producing new ones.

Methotrexate comes under the heading of *antimetabolites,* which trick malignant cells into assimilating them, then impede their growth and division. And prednisone belongs to yet another class of chemotherapy drugs, *steroid compounds,* containing cancer-inhibiting hormones. A fifth category, *tumoricidal antibiotics,* includes the widely used drug doxorubicin.

"This is the standard protocol," Dr. Burgert said. "But we could also give Jason a drug called daunomycin [generically known as daunorubicin], which has been found effective against leukemia. It's being used now in a study on kids with Burkitt's." In other words, while the drug itself was not experimental, the application was. He was offering us participation in a *clinical trial,* also referred to as a *research protocol.*

Through clinical-trial studies doctors evaluate sophisticated new cancer treatments believed superior to existing ones. According to Dr. Smithson, the five-drug protocol for Burkitt's was "the best available at the time," drawn up by the Children's Cancer Study Group. A network of pediatric cancer centers, the CCSG operates under the auspices of the National Cancer Institute, pooling and conferring on test results.

Exploratory drugs are tested in three phases. Phase one, for determining toxicity levels and optimum dosages, relies on volunteers with advanced disease. In 1986 my father was given just months to live. His prostate cancer, diagnosed late, had metastasized extensively to the bone, inflicting excruciating pain. Having witnessed Jason's two-year ordeal, he told us, "At my age don't ask me to do what Jason did, lose my hair and be sick to my stomach all the time. But," he declared, "I'm not done yet."

Dad enlisted in a phase-one study that called for daily injections designed to starve the cancer of the male hormones it feeds on. As of this writing he is still alive and remarkably active for a man his age, cancer or no cancer. And the dosage of leuprolide acetate, now a standard prostate-cancer therapy, has been refined so that he has to take it only once a month.

If phase one proves successful, the knowledge accumulated is incorporated into phase two, which measures the drug's potency against different cancers. Phase three, the study proposed for Jason, compares the new and standard treatments.

"It takes years for agents to take their place in the whole of treatment," notes Dr. Burgert. In the late 1940s methotrexate was first used to treat acute leukemia in children. Even more than forty years later "there are situations," he says, "where the best uses of methotrexate are still being identified."

Jason's doctors went on to outline the benefits of clinical trials, saying that they offered the most up-to-date care and were formulated under strict scientific methods. Most are federally funded and/or regulated and approved by a safety review board. But, they cautioned, experimental treatments come with no guarantee of improved results and are not without unanticipated risks.

For instance daunomycin had damaged the heart muscles of some young Burkitt's patients, especially when used in conjunction with radiation. Each treatment can amplify the other's potential side effects. Alarmed, I asked, "What good is it if we cure our son of cancer, only to have him die of a heart attack?"

Dr. Burgert replied, "We'll monitor Jason very, very closely and conduct regular cardiac tests so that we can note the earliest indication of heart-muscle changes and avoid a serious progression of damage by stopping the daunomycin." He added that we could refuse any research for any reason and could quit the study at any time. Should we decide to withdraw our consent, he assured us, our son's standard treatment would in no way suffer.

Craig and I barely deliberated. We were willing—and, I have to say, desperate enough—to try anything that might help Jason, no matter how slight the gains. You may wince at the idea of your child being used as a guinea pig, which in effect he is. But when our six-year-old's doctors suggested the experimental program, it occurred to me that in the past others faced this same dilemma and said yes. Thanks to them the physicians could hold out hope to us instead of having to say, "I'm sorry, Mr. and Mrs. Gaes, but there's nothing we can do."

We felt privileged to have our son take part in a study that could alter the course of treatment. Jason's protocol is now incorporated into a computerized data base. Physicians contemplating this treatment for Burkitt's patients can punch up his name and see exactly which drugs were given to him and how. And of course the glorious results.

A two-page "Consent to Participation in Medical Research Study" form clarified the protocol's pros and cons, with one disquieting paragraph detailing the possible toxic reactions. "Although unlikely," it read, "the side effects could be life-threatening." Jason and I both signed the document, ostensibly extending "informed consent," an unrealistic concept if there ever was one. Under the circumstances few parents or patients are truly able to make informed decisions, regardless of explicit forms and candid explanations from their doctors.

The National Cancer Institute suggests asking the following questions before entering a young patient in a clinical trial:

- Why is this study being conducted?
- Who has reviewed and approved it?
- Who is sponsoring it? The National Cancer Institute? A major cancer center?
- What are the credentials of its investigators and personnel?
- What information or results is it based on?
- How are patient safety and the study data monitored?
- What are the possible benefits?
- Why is the treatment in this study believed to surpass that currently being used? Why may it not be any better?
- How long will my child be in the study?
- What tests and treatments are involved?
- Will she be hospitalized?
- What are the new treatment's possible side effects or risks?
- How could the study affect my child's daily life?
- Does the study include long-term follow-up care?
- What are our other treatment options, including standard treatment? How do they compare in terms of possible outcomes, reactions, time involved, and quality of life?
- What happens with the results of this study?

Other, extremely important questions to ask concern cost, surely the last thing on your mind at this terrible time. You should know that the government underwrites some experimental treatments, but not all. Not Jason's daunomycin, for example, despite his belonging to a CCSG study group. Medical insurers frequently don't cover these therapies, something we learned firsthand with my father.

In 1986 leuprolide acetate was so new that Medicare had never even heard of it and rejected Dad's claim. A month's prescription cost him

$710. Only after the drug was approved did Medicare pay for it, though not retroactively. It seems an unjust policy to me, penalizing patients who in essence are voluntarily performing a public service.

In any case be sure to ask:

- What are the *total* costs for this therapy?
- Which costs of treatment, if any, are free of charge?
- Which costs must be paid for by us and/or our insurer?
- Does insurance generally pay for this care?
- How successful have you been in getting all costs for this therapy reimbursed by insurers? What is your experience with our insurer?

(For more about contesting disputed insurance claims, see Chapter Nine.)

Learning About Clinical Trials in Your Area

We feel fortunate to have taken our son to a state-of-the-art research center like the Mayo Clinic, where his oncology team was keenly aware of existing protocols for Burkitt's patients. But doctors at all levels of facilities can learn about the over 1,300 experimental programs being conducted nationwide by calling the Physicians Data Query.

You, too, can call (800) 4-CANCER to receive a printout describing ongoing clinical trials in your region or anywhere in the country. These include not only National Cancer Institute studies but those administered by local medical facilities. The NCI estimates that if more physicians utilized the PDQ, the U.S. cancer survival rate would rise 10 percent, saving forty thousand lives annually.

What if your child's doctor doesn't suggest participating in a clinical trial? She might genuinely feel that those available don't promise any significant advantages over the standard therapy. Or your youngster might not meet the very specific and necessary medical qualifications. However, some physicians inadequately inform their patients about research protocols because, quite simply, these experimental programs demand increased paperwork, laboratory work, and so on.

Your doctor is obligated to apprise you and your child of all credible treatment options. Should you suspect that her ambivalence toward clinical trials isn't solely motivated by medical reasoning, make inquiries of the PDQ yourself. Once you've looked over the material, if you want to pursue the matter, obtain a second opinion elsewhere.

Suggested Reading About Clinical Trials
From the National Cancer Institute (800-4-CANCER):

• "What Are Clinical Trials All About?"

A Chemotherapy Session

Chemotherapy may be carried out in a hospital room, outpatient clinic, doctor's office, even at home, although many physicians prefer hospitalizing young patients their first time, as our son was, in order to monitor reactions to the drugs. From observing the number and severity of side effects experienced, the oncologist adjusts and refines the dosage.

Most of Jason's treatments took place at the Mayo Clinic, but also at our pediatrician's office and Worthington Regional Hospital beginning in the fall. His drug schedule alternated so that he received the cyclophosphamide and the methotrexate spinal-fluid treatment in Rochester, after which I gave him the oral prednisone at home for several days. The next week Dr. Faul intravenously dispensed the vincristine, daunomycin, and methotrexate I'd brought home with us.

Whatever the setting the routine varied little. Mornings began with blood and urine tests. By analyzing blood samples, doctors can track the growth or shrinkage of tumors, which release proteins into the blood. Generally speaking, the lower the protein level, the smaller the tumor, and vice versa. Then it was on to radiology, where sonograms and either CAT scans or X rays were taken and studied for any unusual growths.

A full physical examination always followed. The physician felt my son's lymph glands for lumps or swelling, checked his eyes and ears, noted his blood pressure, and took his temperature. All the while we discussed Jason's general health since the previous appointment, his response to the medications, and so forth.

By then the doctor had received the blood test results, which are critical for deciding whether a patient is medically fit for treatment. One potential risk from chemotherapy is suppression of the bone marrow's production of platelets, red cells, and, in particular, white cells, predisposing youngsters to infection. Radiation, too, can ravage white cells. Therefore blood tests may be performed before those sessions as well, to determine if the X-ray dosage should be modified.

Almost every drug therapy conducted in Worthington was postponed because Jason's levels of white cells had dropped precipitously from the cyclophosphamide administered the previous time. If the white count is extremely low, your child's doctor may order an intravenous infusion of antibiotics to ward off infection.

I remember weeks when we had to return to the local blood lab two or three mornings in a row, waiting for Jason's white count to creep back up into a safe range. Then, depending on the rotation, either he received his medicines right there or off we went to Rochester. You can imagine how on those days I appreciated having chemotherapy available locally. Otherwise we would have had to commute across the state or check into a motel for nights on end.

Once Jason's oncologist declared him ready, we were sent to the Mayo's twelfth-floor chemotherapy wing. Some hospitals herd up to three kids into the same cramped room for intravenous treatments, hardly the most sensitive of arrangements. Young patients deserve privacy. Not only do the drugs often induce sickness, but therapy can last hours. Jason would spend three hours tethered to an I.V. pole when being given his cyclophosphamide; *eight* hours when receiving the vincristine, daunomycin, and methotrexate.

The setup on 12A is as thoughtfully designed as any I've seen. A nurses' station sits in the middle of the floor, surrounded by over two dozen private rooms. Most are outfitted with hospital beds, whereas at Dr. Faul's Jason had to lie on an examination table for all eight hours, an uncomfortable setting for a child feeling ill, bored, and cranky.

The Mayo's soothing, cream-colored chemotherapy rooms are decorated with paintings and posters, anything to make them as cheery as possible. One wall poster depicts Garfield, the heavy-lidded comic-strip cat, imploring, fittingly, "Why me?" Jason always crossed his fingers that he'd get a room with a television set, which helped us pass the time. Treatment may be administered once per week, once per month, or five days in a row for a number of weeks or months. The schedule depends on your child's type of cancer, the drugs prescribed, and how his body responds.

Methods of Administering Chemotherapy

Chemotherapy is delivered to the bloodstream via one of three main paths:

• **Orally.**   Many drugs are available in ingestible liquid, capsule, or tablet form. They enter the blood through the lining of the stomach or upper intestines. For instance Jason's prednisone came as tiny white, beige, or pink pills. Not all anticancer medicines can be taken by mouth, however, because they either damage the stomach lining or aren't readily absorbed.

• **Intramuscularly (I.M.).**   Some agents must seep gradually into the bloodstream to be effective. These are injected into a muscle in the arm, thigh, or buttocks, like a standard flu shot, and take no more than fifteen seconds or so. Of the more common pediatric chemotherapy drugs, only bleomycin, used to manage squamous-cell carcinoma, Hodgkin's disease, and non-Hodgkin's lymphomas, is given this way.

• **Intravenously.**   The most prevalent and fastest means of introducing chemotherapeutic drugs into the bloodstream is directly through the veins. Doctors either inject the chemicals using a syringe *(I.V. push)* or insert the hollow needle, then infuse the medicine slowly *(I.V. drip)* from a plastic bag hanging from a portable metal pole. Before chemo commences, a liquid sedative and antinausea medicine are often administered to blunt adverse reactions, as are fluids for flushing the drugs through the system.

Since a child's veins are small, piercing the vein requires the special skills of a pediatric chemotherapy nurse. When all goes smoothly, says Jason, "The I.V. hurts for only a split second." It didn't distress him as much if he didn't see the needle, he claimed, preferring to bury his face against me. The drugs were infused into the back of my son's hand, but your child's chemotherapist may select other sites.

An accomplished nurse knows to "open" the vein first by either lightly tapping or slapping the area, or wrapping it with a warm cloth or compress. To steady Jason's hand, some taped it to a board for support; others didn't bother. We were fortunate to have a chemotherapy nurse administer the drugs virtually every time. But I know of instances where a less experienced hospital intern or resident has taken up to ten tries to insert the I.V. needle, resulting in one hysterical child and two upset parents. As Craig will attest, "stickings" can be difficult to sit through.

Once at Saint Marys my husband sat with Jason as a student doctor clumsily tried putting the I.V. into his hand. Our six-year-old, normally a brave little patient, started screaming, "Stop! It hurts! It hurts!" but the woman kept jabbing away.

Craig is shy by nature, but after watching her do this five or six times, he finally exploded. "Enough is enough!" he protested. "You're not going to practice on him anymore." As I recall, some packing-house language followed. "This isn't a guinea pig you're working on," my husband fumed, "this is a child. You tried, you couldn't do it, so now *she's* going to do it." He pointed at the instructor, who, without saying a word, took over and effortlessly slipped the needle into the vein on the first attempt.

I realize interns must train somewhere, but it just seems that I.V. stickings can be traumatic enough for young people without subjecting them to excessive torment. If you arrive at your child's appointment and don't find an intravenous specialist present, specify that you want an expert to perform the insertion. Unless absolutely no chemotherapy nurses are available, medical centers will usually accommodate your request.

The drugs may seep out of the vein while being pushed or infused, causing an acute burning sensation and/or *hematoma,* a swelling of the skin. This occurred several times when Jason received his vincristine. He used to howl with pain. A nurse would wrap his hand in hot towels, the heat dilating the blood vessels so that the medicine could flow more freely. Eventually the searing feeling would subside. If you observe redness or swelling around the I.V. site, alert your youngster's doctor or nurse immediately.

Weeks or months of constant sticking gradually deplete the number of healthy veins. After a while Jason's nurses had to switch to his other hand. Sometimes so many veins "blow," or collapse, that vessels in the legs, scalp, or big toe must be utilized. In the event that all the veins suffer damage, your child's doctor may resort to cutting into a wrist for a usable vein, an incisional procedure requiring anesthesia.

Nowadays new methods of administering chemotherapy spare young patients unpleasant insertions and complications. Under local anesthesia a flexible plastic tube called a *right-atrial catheter* (also known as a Broviac-Hickman, Cook, or Leonard catheter) is surgically implanted into a large vein in the upper chest, where it can remain for up to two

years as a permanent intravenous line. Instead of having to thread a
new vein each time, the medical team feeds the drugs into the tube's
top, which protrudes from the chest. Then they cap it and tape the
visible portion securely in place. Underneath regular clothes it is not
even noticeable.

Most of the pediatric-cancer patients we met preferred this device to
repeated stickings. But when Jason's doctors proposed the idea, our son
wouldn't hear of it. An avid swimmer, he felt it would interfere with one
of the few athletic activities he could still enjoy. Treatment choices for
cancer patients are few and far between, so Craig and I decided we'd
go along with whatever Jason wanted. And, I must admit, at the time
I felt a bit intimidated by the amount of care the catheter required.

In retrospect my reservations were unwarranted. A nurse or doctor
will show you how to flush out the device, clean the area, and change
dressings, all simple daily procedures. Another option is the implanta-
tion of a small pump that releases the chemotherapy continuously, and
in greater concentration, to either the area of the tumor or directly to
the malignant tissue itself.

• Chemotherapy may also be injected just beneath the skin's surface
(subcutaneously, or *SC);* into an artery *(intra-arterially);* into the abdomen
or the lung's pleural cavity *(intracavitarily);* or into the spinal fluid *(intrathetically,* or *IT).* Dr. Smithson used the latter route to deliver Jason's
methotrexate every other week, something our son feared more than a
pop quiz in school. In Chapter Two we described the lumbar puncture,
or spinal tap, for withdrawing cerebrospinal fluid. It became a two-stage
procedure. With the syringe still in our son's back, Dr. Smithson emp-
tied the middle cylinder of the fluid, replaced it with the chemotherapeutic drugs, injected them through the cylinder, and then
removed the whole apparatus.

Suggested Reading About Chemotherapy
(For parents and young patients)

From the National Cancer Institute (800-4-CANCER):
• "Chemotherapy & You/A Guide to Self-Help During Treatment"

CHAPTER FIVE

SHORT-TERM SIDE EFFECTS OF RADIATION AND CHEMOTHERAPY

Coping with Hair Loss • Ways to Manage Adverse Reactions • Controlling Infection

Sitting and waiting for my son's chemotherapy or radiation treatments, I'd glance around at the gaunt, bald boys and girls playing and laughing together and think to myself, *We don't belong here.* Jason, never sick a day in his life until now, still looked like Jason: golden-haired, pink-cheeked, bright-eyed—a healthy kid, not one with cancer.

It was denial of course. I would quickly come to realize that we belonged among those children more than I wanted to admit.

Because we'd missed our family vacation to Kansas City, Craig and I promised the kids that when he came to Rochester on the weekend, we'd go to Valley Fair, a Minneapolis amusement park an hour and a half away.

On the drive north that drizzly Sunday we stopped to buy camera film. It's funny: I'd never been a shutterbug before. Now I suddenly felt compelled to photograph Jason at every opportunity, fearing, I suppose, that he might not be alive much longer.

While waiting in the van for me, Craig began to comb our son's hair, which stuck out at all angles from the rain. To my husband's shock a bunch came off in his hand. When I climbed back in with the film, Craig's grim expression told me something was wrong.

"Look," he said, rubbing Jason's head and displaying the fistful of blond hair.

HANDLING HAIR LOSS

That was only the beginning. Between the cranial radiation and the chemotherapy, within a matter of weeks Jason was as bald as a cueball, with the bright red X's applied for radiation making his scalp look like a tic-tac-toe board. When we'd raised the possibility that he might lose his hair from treatment, our six-year-old cried inconsolably—though, as it turned out, not at the prospect of baldness per se.

"I had blond hair but thought my scalp underneath was *brown*," Jason recalls, laughing. "That's what I worried about, walking around with a brown head!" Our advice to parents is to discuss this and other potential side effects with young patients, not to alarm them but to prepare them. Kids, blessed with overactive imaginations, are likely to envision consequences more awful than the reality, as Jason did.

Encouraging him to express his fears enabled Craig and me to reassure our son that, no, he would not be left with a chocolate-colored head. Throughout his illness Jason continually surprised us with his desire to know what to expect. We answered him as sensitively and honestly as we knew how, using concepts and language he could grasp.

Hair loss, or *alopecia,* is a common side effect of chemotherapy and skull irradiation. Both treatments interfere with rapidly generating cells, whether normal or abnormal. With their extremely high rate of cellular turnover, hair follicles are vulnerable anywhere on the body: skull, eyebrows, eyelashes, pubic area, arms, armpits, legs, chest.

Will your child's hair fall out? One determinant is the chemotherapy drugs themselves. For example, two of the five prescribed for Jason, prednisone and methotrexate, are not known to cause this condition, while vincristine, daunomycin, and cyclophosphamide frequently do. Then, too, patients' reactions vary, even to the same medication. Not every youngster on cyclophosphamide loses her hair, and those that do may experience loss ranging from mild to severe. At the Mayo Clinic we met children whose hair came out in clumps over a period of days. Others' fell out gradually over weeks.

Before chemotherapy begins, ask your child's oncologist about experimental methods of curtailing or preventing hair loss. A *scalp tourniquet,* made of cloth, is wrapped tightly around the head just prior to treatment and left there until about fifteen minutes afterward. The purpose of the band is to constrict blood flow to the scalp and block high concentrations of the drugs from reaching the follicles.

Another device, called a *cold cap,* employs *hypothermia.* Essentially an ice pack, it, too, is placed on the patient's head before drugs are administered. The scalp's blood vessels contract from the cold, so that less medicine gets through to the follicles. While the cold cap has been found effective for some patients, it doesn't work for everyone, sometimes producing headaches or patchy hair loss that ultimately looks less attractive than full baldness.

Again, discuss these with your physician. Many strongly oppose any technique that would prevent medication from entering the scalp. According to the National Cancer Institute, hypothermia should never be used on lymphoma or leukemia sufferers, or anyone with a cancer that might metastasize to the scalp.

Putting the problem of hair loss in perspective, it is a comparatively minor inconvenience that doesn't affect a child's health and isn't painful. Still, the first question young patients often ask upon learning they have cancer is, "Will my hair fall out?"

Certainly the psychological trauma isn't as great for small children as for adolescents, whose appearance is so entwined with their self-image. Hairstyles represent one of a teenager's few means of self-expression, perhaps even more so now than in our generation's day. To lose their locks at that age is like losing their voice. As for girls, in a society that associates a gorgeous head of hair with femininity, this upsetting consequence can deflate their self-esteem for a time.

Young patients' feelings of distress are perfectly normal and are attributable to more than mere vanity. A bald head is a terrifying symbol of a body out of control. In addition it proclaims to others, *I have cancer. I'm different.* As you'll no doubt recall from your own youth, during this confusing time of life teenagers want nothing more than to fit in. So while overall losing one's hair isn't the end of the world, we don't want to diminish its very real psychological impact on youngsters.

I have to admit, at first the sight of Jason's bald head sent a shiver up my spine. I couldn't delude myself, even for a moment, that no life-threatening illness lurked within his body. But as with many other troubling aspects of this disease, both patients and parents come to accept hair loss as a trade-off for a possible cure, and that seems a fair exchange. Also, as we frequently reminded our young son, with the cessation of aggressive treatment the hair usually comes back. If the drugs and/or irradiation have done what they're supposed to, hopefully the cancer does not.

Jason adapted to his baldness fairly quickly, thanks to the influence of his buddy Harlan, a teenager suffering from soft-tissue sarcoma. We met Harlan and his mother at Rochester's Ronald McDonald House (then known as Northland House), where we were all staying. Harlan, from Wabash, Indiana, had recently undergone minor surgery to re-place a chemotherapy chest catheter.

Despite the twelve years' difference in their ages, Harlan and Jason became fast friends. My son absolutely idolized the older boy, whose hair had fallen out some time before. "He was eighteen, but he seemed real grown up," Jason recalls. "Even though he knew he might not make it, he was always very upbeat and positive." Harlan accepted his baldness good-naturedly, and this improved Jason's outlook about his own appearance.

As August approached, only a few dozen scraggly hairs still topped our six-year-old's head. One morning the two of us attended a church near the Mayo Clinic. Normally we walked down the aisle to the pews in front, but this time Jason insisted, "If I can't sit in back, I'm not going in." He was convinced that everyone would point and stare at him like he was some sort of weirdo: the Little Boy with the Bald Head. His embarrassment deeply concerned me.

Then Harlan got a hold of him. He took Jason to a Rochester shopping mall, and as they ambled out of a store, the teenager com-manded, "Look around you." Jason complied. "Do you see anybody staring at you?"

"No."

"Of course not," Harlan said, smiling. He convinced Jason that baldness wasn't something to be ashamed of, it was a badge of courage. "Seeing how comfortable Harlan was with his baldness really helped me a lot," Jason says. "I realized that not everyone would laugh at me. Maybe they'd even think having a bald head was cool."

Our son grew to feel so much at ease that Craig used to kiddingly call him skinhead and make wisecracks like "Hey, watch that head; the sun's glaring in my eyes!" No one laughed louder than Jason. We abandoned thoughts of buying him a wig, one option for those unhappy with their appearance. Harlan occasionally wore a hairpiece, though with typical self-deprecating humor he used to put it on backward or stuff it down his shirt for a laugh.

Forty percent of body heat escapes through the head. Not surprisingly many young patients complain that the wigs feel hot and itchy. In our experience most boys eventually did without hairpieces, either donning hats or going au natural. For obvious reasons girls usually have more difficulty adjusting to hair loss. About half of those we met preferred wigs to scarves, turbans, or hats.

If your child thinks she'd feel more confident in a wig, it's a good idea to obtain one before treatment starts. This way she can get used to wearing and being seen in it as she's losing her hair. Some hairpieces look so natural, friends and classmates may never suspect the patient is bald underneath, only that she's changed her hairstyle.

While parents should certainly assist and support youngsters who choose this alternative, you don't want to inadvertently contribute to feelings of self-consciousness. Explain that wearing a wig is fine if it makes a person feel good about himself, but baldness needn't be hidden from others. I advocate encouraging children to be as candid as possible about their condition.

To find a wig retailer, look under "Hair Replacements, Goods and Supplies" in your local yellow pages. Some specialize in replacement hair for cancer patients, offering private fittings. Synthetic wigs may not look as authentic as those made of human hair, but they are cooler, easier to care for, and less expensive.

Insurers often cover wig purchases due to medical problems. If yours doesn't, the cost is tax-deductible. However, many hospitals loan hairpieces free of charge. Your facility's social worker can tell you more about this. The American Cancer Society, too, offers wigs to cancer patients as a free service. Arrange for an appointment by calling your regional ACS office at (800) ACS-2345.

Instead of a wig, we bought our son a closetful of caps representing each of his favorite sports teams. He must have had one for nearly every franchise in North America, with jerseys and T-shirts to match: basketball's Boston Celtics, football's Los Angeles Raiders, and, not wanting to appear disloyal, our Minnesota Twins baseball team.

Unbeknown to me at first, Jason became so casual about his baldness that he stopped wearing them. Upon his return to school later that year, he and Tim left the house together every morning and as soon as they rounded the corner, Jason took off his cap and handed it to his eager twin. The boys were in the same first-grade class. At my first parent-teacher conference their teacher remarked to me, "I don't know if you're aware of this, Mrs. Gaes, but it's against school policy for students to wear hats in the classroom."

I felt my blood pressure rise. "Gee," I replied, "I just thought that wearing a hat would make Jason feel more comfortable."

"Jason?" she said, perplexed. "I'm talking about *Tim*. He says you told him he had to wear it all day!"

Today Jason recalls, "Sometimes I liked to play games with my baldness. Tim sat behind me in science class. One time I felt something rubbing against the back of my head. 'Tim, what are you doing?' I asked. '*Shhh,*' he whispered, 'just look straight ahead.'

"He drew a face on the back of my head—eyes, mouth, nose, hair—then put my cap on me backward. That way I could turn around in my seat and talk to my brother while still 'facing' the teacher. All the other kids started giggling. Even the teacher had to laugh once she realized what was going on."

Being bald also won Jason first prize for best costume at a Halloween party. No, he didn't go as Telly Savalas, but as menacing Mr. T, since relegated to the abandoned closet of Youngsters' Erstwhile TV Favorites. We draped chains around his neck and glued on a black mohawk, beard, and mustache, so that he looked just like the scowling member of the then hugely popular A-Team. Jason didn't want to go at first but wound up coming home with a bagful of audio cassettes. The emcee who handed him his prize remarked to the crowd, "Anybody that would shave his head for a Halloween costume *deserves* to win!"

OTHER POTENTIAL SHORT-TERM SIDE EFFECTS OF TREATMENT AND WAYS TO MANAGE THEM

Improved technology and technique enable modern radiotherapists to give patients higher, more accurate doses of radiation, while reducing the severity of side effects. But despite precautions such as lead shields and blocks, inevitably a number of radiosensitive normal cells are damaged or destroyed, and adverse reactions occur. These cells may sit near the target site or a good distance away.

Likewise, although today's chemotherapeutic drugs afford patients optimum potency with a minimum of side effects, numerous physical and/or emotional problems may result. I'll always remember the stark analogy Dr. Bringelsen drew for us at the start of treatment.

"These drugs are poison," she said frankly. "At the same time that we're poisoning cancer cells, we're poisoning good cells. So we poison Jason to the point where his body can't take any more, nurse him back to health, then poison him again."

The following pages describe the more common potential side effects of both radiation and chemotherapy. We've combined them, as there is much overlap. Those exclusive to one form of treatment are indicated as such. A chart at the back of this chapter lists the consequences of the medications frequently used to fight pediatric cancer, classifying their side effects according to medical urgency.

I must warn you, it makes for disturbing reading. Some drugs have potentially dozens of unwanted side effects that range from the relatively minor, such as diarrhea, fatigue, or appetite loss, to the potentially serious, such as hallucinations, convulsions, or hearing loss. The danger of kidney or liver damage always exists, a situation your child's doctor will monitor through blood tests and urinalysis.

We emphasize that these are *potential* side effects. Your child may experience many, several, or none at all. Or he may suffer a bothersome side effect after one treatment but not after another. For example, some children become nauseous or vomit from radiation, yet those treatments never made Jason sick. There's no telling how your child will react. The good news is that in most instances the side effects are reversible, ceasing once therapy is completed or soon thereafter.

Parents must be aware of all possible side effects in order to recognize and report unanticipated symptoms to the doctor at once. If your child reacts poorly to the prescription or to radiation, his physician may modify the dosage and extend the treatment period. A lower dose of medication or irradiation in no way decreases a treatment's effectiveness or a patient's chances for recovery. *Never,* however, discontinue a drug without consulting your doctor.

Have your physician list for you the possible adverse reactions. You may also want to look up the drugs and their side effects in the *Physicians' Desk Reference,* found in the reference section of most public libraries. It can also be purchased from any major bookstore. Easier to comprehend is *Advice for the Patient: Drug Information in Lay Language,* published by the United States Phamacopeial Convention and available in hospital and medical libraries.

As for informing young patients about side effects, we told Jason only about those that might occur right away, such as hair loss and vomiting. With his life in peril, we didn't see any point in bringing up long-term hazards, such as infertility and intellectual impairment.

Ask your youngster's doctor the following questions:

• *Are there any medications my child should not take while under treatment?* No matter how seemingly innocuous the product, whether prescription or over-the-counter, get your physician's approval before giving your child *any* medicine, including vitamins, antacids, sleeping pills, nose sprays, antihistamines, cough medicine, antibiotics, laxatives, or aspirin. The latter, for example, can stimulate bleeding in patients taking prednisone or dexamethasone. Instead buy aspirin-free pain relievers, generically known as acetaminophen.

• *Must my child avoid certain foods?* According to the National Cancer Institute patients on procarbazine should stay away from foods containing tyramine, usually found in products aged to enhance their flavor: cheese, yogurt, sour cream, pickled herring, chicken liver, canned figs, raisins, bananas, avocados, soy sauce, fava beans, yeast extracts, and tenderized meats. Any of these can provoke a dangerous reaction.

• *Which immunizations can my child safely receive?* "Live virus" vaccines for measles, German measles, rubella, mumps, and some polio, are potentially harmful to youngsters receiving certain medications and should be postponed until after treatment. Other, non-live-virus shots may be permitted, but always consult your physician first.

(Note: Many of these side effects can spoil a child's appetite. Solutions to radiation- and chemotherapy-related eating problems are covered in Chapter Eight.)

Nausea and Vomiting

Except for children getting radiation to the head or abdomen, nausea and vomiting are more likely to accompany chemotherapy. Within hours of his first I.V., Jason became progressively sicker. Watching over him was like awaiting an impending storm looming on the horizon. "It's starting," I overheard someone whisper from the hall.

Strangely I felt almost relieved when the rising waves of nausea and vomiting came on, like, *Thank God, the chemotherapy is doing what it's supposed to.* I now know that there is no relation between the severity or mildness of side effects and the medicine's effectiveness.

Nausea and vomiting may begin anywhere from two to six hours after chemotherapy is administered, lasting a few hours or up to several days. My son tolerated the vincristine-daunomycin-methotrexate treatments given in Worthington fairly well, but the cyclophosphamide knocked him for a loop. We usually returned home from Rochester around nine in the evening. Like clockwork at midnight Jason would start throwing up roughly every fifteen minutes. The next day, every thirty minutes, until by late afternoon it tapered off, and he felt well enough to sit up on the sofa. Two or three days typically passed before he was able to nibble on food again and attend school, a pattern that continued throughout treatment.

One way to alleviate discomfort is to have chemotherapy delivered late in the day so that your child can sleep through the sickness as much as possible. Another is for him to be given *antiemetic* (antinausea) medicine, although doctors prefer avoiding this with young children. Jason's doctors prescribed two powerful liquid controllers called Phenergan and Benadryl, which he swallowed about an hour beforehand. The pharmacy flavored the Phenergan lemon-lime, ostensibly to make it more palatable, but Jason could not stomach the taste. I think he dreaded it as much if not more than the chemotherapy itself. Today if I make lemon or lime Kool-Aid, he gags at the mere smell.

Antiemetic drugs do not always work. To help quell nausea and vomiting nonmedically, try flat ginger ale, tea, sucking candies, soda, bouillon, crackers, or plain chicken, but avoid milk products, which are harder to digest. Some youngsters are so sensitive that even being in a particular place—a hospital room, the car, a cooking area—may induce vomiting. The National Cancer Institute suggests these ways to make patients comfortable:

- Loosen tight, constrictive clothing.
- Remove any traces of vomit, such as stained clothes or bed linens.
- Make sure the room is quiet and well ventilated.
- Periodically dab your child's face with a cool, damp washcloth.
- To get rid of the unpleasant taste, have your youngster rinse out her mouth with cool water or mouthwash, or use a damp cloth or swab to gently wipe her mouth and tongue.
- Help her find a comfortable position, with the head slightly elevated.
- Encourage her to take deep breaths and concentrate on how she will feel once the sickness subsides—anything to divert attention from the nausea.
- Do what you can to eliminate cooking odors, for chemotherapy agents can sharpen a patient's sense of smell. Some nights following Jason's drug therapy I used to ask Craig to take Adam, Tim, and Missy out to eat, because kitchen aromas just set Jason's stomach churning.

If vomiting persists, children run the risk of dehydration, or an excessive loss of body fluid and crucial minerals. Excessive sweating from fever or diarrhea can also cause it. If any of these conditions continues for more than a day or two, or is especially severe, notify your child's doctor immediately. This can be a life-threatening emergency.

Fatigue

Jason's radiation appointments left him utterly drained. Afterward we'd go back to Northland House. While most of the kids there frolicked on the jungle gym outside, my son hardly had the strength to sit up. He mainly spent his days lying on a sofa, watching TV. One weekend he wanted us to take him shopping. No sooner did we enter the mall than

Jason panted, "Mom, I can't walk any farther." Craig and I had to push our six-year-old around in a rented baby stroller that he barely fit into, his feet dangling over the sides.

Exactly why radiation and chemotherapy patients frequently suffer fatigue is unclear. Two probable factors are the dissolving malignant cells—"tumor garbage," in Dr. Gilchrist's words—that mount up in the blood, depleting energy. Drinking several quarts of fluids a day helps dispose of these waste products. In addition the body has to work overtime to replenish the damaged healthy cells.

If your child tires easily, encourage him to rest. Schedule intermittent naps throughout the day, limit visitors, and cut back on—but don't cut out—activities. As we explain in Chapter Seven, while it's important for kids with cancer to live as normally as possible, they must learn to listen to their bodies, which will dictate sensible limits. This lethargy can outlast treatment incidentally. It wasn't until a full month after his final radiation session that Jason began to display his former vitality. Craig notes dryly that the exhaustion seemed mysteriously to recur whenever he asked our son to perform some household chore.

Sore Mouth, Gums, or Throat

All things considered, Jason got through radiation with minimal problems. Well over a week after he finished treatment, however, I brought him back to the Mayo Clinic for chemotherapy. During the routine physical exam Dr. Smithson wanted to know about any unusual symptoms since our previous appointment.

"Well," I said worriedly, "Jason hardly ate enough to keep a bird alive."

"Sore throat?" he immediately asked Jason, who nodded. The doctor didn't appear surprised, since patients receiving radiation to the head and neck sometimes experience soreness or burning that begins days to weeks after treatment. Most chemotherapeutic drugs can also bring about this delayed condition. But when Dr. Smithson peered into my son's mouth, he exclaimed, "Oh my!"

Jason's inner cheeks, gums, and palate were full of radiation blisters, which would soon peel until the tissue hung down in sheets. Tears welled in my eyes; I felt like a negligent mother. Why hadn't I noticed this before? Dr. Smithson said gently, "Geralyn, how would you know to look there if Jason didn't complain?" Which he didn't. He never mentioned that his mouth hurt. He just seemed to have no appetite, another common side effect of chemotherapy.

Dr. Smithson prescribed an anesthetic mouthwash to soothe the ulcerated skin. The National Cancer Institute recommends giving this to children at least one hour before meals, as the numbing effect may suppress the normal gag reflex and heighten the risk of choking. Anesthetic ointments, for applying directly to the sore, and ice chips also provide relief. My son used to pop them into his mouth regularly like sucking candy. Another remedy, for older children, is to swab or rinse their mouths with hydrogen peroxide and warm water, a mixture that should be spit out, *never* swallowed.

The burns, combined with the weakness, made eating a chore. Over the next several weeks Jason lost fifteen pounds from his already skinny forty-five-pound frame. It's wise during this time to refrain from serving spicy or coarse foods, which can further irritate the mouth and are painful to swallow. One trick to ease uncomfortable swallowing is to have your child tilt his head either back or forward.

Thick Saliva or Dry Mouth

Radiation to the head and neck and some drugs may affect the salivary glands so that they produce either thick saliva or very little. The former nuisance is treatable by rinsing with club soda. Most drugstores stock nonprescription artificial saliva preparations with names such as Moistir and Glandosane, which help dilute the spittle and cleanse the mouth.

Jason developed dry mouth, or *xerostomia*. For a while I watched in astonishment as he guzzled glass after glass of water. Several times a day we gave him ice chips and sugarless lozenges and chewing gum to moisten his mouth. Your child's doctor can recommend a saline solution like those mentioned above, glycerine swabs, or a mouthwash. However, avoid brands containing alcohol, which only exacerbates the dryness. Placing a humidifier in your child's bedroom may help too.

Because saliva protects teeth from decay, reduced flow can lead to serious dental problems. Maintaining proper oral hygiene is more complicated when children with low platelet counts must refrain from using water-jet devices, hard-bristle or electric toothbrushes, and floss—anything that might induce bleeding. A child receiving radiation may even have to have his braces removed until the end of treatment.

If the count is normal, youngsters can floss carefully, and should clean their teeth with an extremely soft brush or cotton swab and a nonabrasive fluoride toothpaste. Your doctor or dentist may suggest a fluoride rinse or gel as well. To clean infants' and toddlers' teeth and gums, use a soft, clean cloth dipped in a solution of one cup cool water and one-quarter teaspoon each of salt and baking soda. Repeat this after every meal.

Although dental work often must be postponed during radiation and chemotherapy, consult regularly with your child's dentist. It's important that an eye be kept on younger children, for radiation can make their teeth develop abnormally. This happened to Jason. The calluses inside his mouth prevented his baby teeth from falling out and the permanent teeth from erupting through the gum as they should. So in 1988, two years after completing treatment, he had to undergo oral surgery, in which the baby teeth and blistered tissue were removed and the new teeth literally yanked down into his mouth.

Altered Taste, Loss of Taste

Along with our son's other mouth-related problems, he experienced a strange, metallic taste, which can occur from both radiation and chemotherapy. Besides further diminishing his already skimpy appetite, "It kind of upset my stomach," says Jason, "but I got used to it." Some children complain of not being able to distinguish flavors at all. Doctors call this condition *mouth blindness*. You can counteract the bad taste by having your child suck on a sourball while undergoing chemotherapy. We never tried this; Jason was usually so sedated, I worried he might accidentally choke on the hard candy. But other patients find it works.

Irritated Skin

Skin is comprised of fast-generating cells sensitive to radiation and chemotherapy, so irradiated areas often turn tender, dry, and flaky. Or the upper layers may shed, leaving the new skin feeling "wet," as if peeled from a sunburn. Kids on chemotherapy can develop rashes or discolored skin along the injected vein. Other, unusual reactions include darkened skin and fingernails, from the drugs cyclophosphamide or doxorubicin, and colored bumps on the fingertips, elbows, or palms, from bleomycin.

Precautionary Measures

• Children receiving radiation should be careful not to irritate the treated area. Throughout therapy and for several weeks after dress your youngster in loose-fitting clothes made of soft, natural fabrics, such as cotton.

• Dispense with potential irritants, such as strong soaps, deodorants, perfume or cologne, powders and lotions, using only those skin-care products suggested by your doctor. Look on the label for "fragrance free" and "hypoallergenic." Radiation therapist Dr. Paula Schomberg of the Mayo Clinic says, "We usually recommend lanolin-based aloe vera creams during treatment."

• Keep kids out of the sun. Radiation patients cannot use sunscreens, so cover their heads with wide-brimmed hats or scarves. Children on methotrexate should also avoid exposure to ultraviolet rays, as the drug intensifies the skin's susceptibility to burning. If the chemotherapy is not accompanied by radiation, use a suntan lotion with a high sun-protection factor, preferably SPF 15 or higher.

• Youngsters who lose their hair from treatment may complain that their heads feel especially sensitive. Try washing the scalp with a mild dandruff shampoo, sprinkling it with cooling cornstarch, or massaging in a little olive oil.

• Extreme hot or cold can further aggravate already damaged skin. Therefore never use hot-water bottles or compresses, ice packs, or heat lamps.

• Boys and girls old enough to shave should put away their manual and electric razors temporarily, unless okayed by the doctor.

• Do not apply bandages or anything adhesive to the skin.

Diarrhea and Constipation

Both chemotherapy and abdominal or pelvic radiation can cause diarrhea, controllable through a low-residue diet. Declare a moratorium on fresh fruit, grains, nuts, raw vegetables, fried food, yogurt, and anything else that has given your child diarrhea in the past. Instead serve cheese, eggs, white rice, and, for restoring lost potassium, lean meat, fish, boiled and mashed potatoes, peach and apricot nectar, and bananas. To prevent dehydration, see that your child drinks lots of fluids. Diarrhea is usually not a serious problem, except in children under three years of age. But should it persist for more than two days, contact your physician, who may prescribe medication.

Vincristine, one of the drugs Jason took, is known to produce stubborn constipation, also correctable through a modified diet. Simply reverse the just-mentioned dietary dos and don'ts. Encourage your child to eat fruits, vegetables, and bran cereals and to drink juice. If that does not work, the doctor may recommend a stool softener or suppository. *Never* give a young chemotherapy patient a laxative or an enema without first consulting your physician.

Another tip for regulating bowel movements is to make sure the patient exercises every day, within the limits recommended by his doctor. Even if he is confined to bed, assist him in flexing his arms, legs, and neck.

Heartburn, Stomachaches
(chemotherapy only)

These side effects sometimes occur in patients taking either prednisone or dexamethasone. To repress heartburn or stomachaches, it helps if the child drinks half a glass of milk or swallows one to two tablespoons of antacid with each dose. Be aware, however, that antacids containing salicylates (the chemical family that includes aspirin) may have the same blood-thinning effect as aspirin. In addition, antacids composed of magnesium hydroxide may cause diarrhea, while those made with aluminum hydroxide or calcium carbonate can constipate. Ask your doctor to recommend a brand for your child.

Round Face, Weight Gain
(chemotherapy only)

Chemotherapeutic steroids such as prednisone have been found to cause fluid retention in the ankles and/or face. At one point during treatment, Jason's head seemed to swell up like a balloon. Plus, prednisone is known to trigger a ravenous appetite. By late summer my son had acquired a potbelly, which looked funny on his otherwise scrawny frame. There's not much that can be done to correct these conditions, except to reduce your child's fat and salt intake. His doctor may also suggest a diuretic for flushing excess water from the body, but never use one without a physician's supervision.

Bloody or Discolored Urine (chemotherapy only)

Jason's doctors warned us that the cyclophosphamide might irritate his bladder, a side effect of other drugs too. That's why it's important for the patient to consume liquids, which accelerate the drugs through her system. Normally on our long drives home from Rochester, I'd pull over to get Jason something to drink. One time, however, he managed to sleep the length of the ride and didn't take in the requisite amount of fluids.

The next morning I heard him holler from the bathroom, "Mom, there's something the matter!" He was urinating blood. *Oh, my God,* I thought, running for the phone, *kidney failure.* To my surprise Dr. Smithson didn't sound terribly alarmed. He calmly explained that the cyclophosphamide had apparently tarried too long in the bladder, resulting in *hemorrhagic cystitis.* "Just give Jason plenty of fluids," was his recommendation. The problem vanished in a matter of days.

Drugs such as daunomycin and doxorubicin can produce red urine for up to two weeks following treatment, and methotrexate, a deep yellow. Plus the odor may seem unusually pungent. While these temporary side effects are not serious, alert the doctor, if only to spare you and your child unnecessary anxiety.

Low Blood Counts

As explained in Chapter Four, cancer treatment frequently suppresses the bone marrow, where most blood components are produced. Before radiation or chemotherapy your child's doctor will monitor his blood's red cells, white cells, and platelets. Deficiencies in these predispose young patients to anemia, infection, and hemorrhaging, respectively. But what about between appointments? What warning signs should parents heed?

A lack of red blood cells deprives a youngster of oxygen, rendering him pale, listless, and out of breath. Other symptoms include headaches, chills, dizziness, and irritability. Usually vitamins and iron supplements are sufficient for maintaining a healthy count. But should full-blown anemia develop, your child's doctor may order a blood transfusion.

Children who exhibit a marked decrease in white blood cells are less resistant to infection. For them an ordinary cold can escalate into a major medical crisis. Symptoms to note and report to the physician include:

• Coughing
• Fever, chills, sweating
• Runny nose
• Sore throat
• Burning or painful urination
• Bloody urine or stool
• Black, tarry stool
• Diarrhea
• Red, swollen areas, warm to the touch
• Lingering sores
• Infections of the eyes, nose, lips, or anus

Antibiotics have proven effective against bacterial infections but not viral illnesses such as chicken pox, in which case treatment may be suspended and other medications prescribed.

Typically sometime after radiation or chemotherapy a youngster's white counts fall, only to rebound naturally in a few days. It is wise during this vulnerable period to quarantine your youngster from anyone with an infectious ailment, such as a cold, flu, measles, mumps, and chicken pox. I can't say I took any extraordinary steps other than to bar Jason from shopping malls, basketball games, and crowded places in general until his counts returned to normal.

You can help ward off infection by: (a) thoroughly cleansing cuts with antiseptic and continuing to do so several times daily until they heal; and (b) taking temperatures orally instead of rectally.

In the event that the white counts fail to bounce back and an infection seems to defy medication, a transfusion of white blood cells may be ordered. Because a closer match is required for white cells than for red, the patient's parents or siblings often act as donors if their blood types are compatible.

Donating from within your family brings peace of mind. Although the odds of contracting the human immunodeficiency virus (HIV) that causes Acquired Immune Deficiency Syndrome (AIDS) from a blood transfusion are low—one in one hundred thousand, according to the U.S. Centers for Disease Control—what parent wants to risk the possibility? As of mid-1991 blood transfusions had infected 255 youngsters with this presently incurable disease.

Due to the absence of clotting cells, children with low platelet counts *(thrombocytopenia)* tend to bruise and bleed easily. Should your child hemorrhage, apply a clean cloth or paper towel to the wound firmly until the bleeding stops. For nose bleeds sit him up and tightly squeeze the bridge of the nose for ten minutes or so. Anytime you cannot control sustained bleeding, call your child's doctor immediately. In addition observe urine and stool for blood, which might indicate internal bleeding.

When the platelet level drops, the minor childhood injuries we normally take for granted become a source of great concern. I used to cut Jason's meat for him at dinner, because even a slight nick could bring on profuse bleeding. Craig and I also discouraged Jason from contact activities, though kids being kids, accidents inevitably happened.

One time Jason tried grabbing a wooden hockey stick away from Tim and got a sliver in his hand. When it was removed, the wound bled and wouldn't stop, until finally a pediatric surgeon had to cauterize it. Similar episodes occurred again and again. Reflecting on that time and those mad dashes to hospital emergency rooms, Craig says wearily, "I sure aged a few years."

Other Side Effects of Radiation

- Earaches and infection from hardened ear wax, usually only if the ears are within the radiation site. Tell your doctor, who may recommend ear drops. Hearing loss is rarely seen in children.
- Dizziness
- Inflammation of irradiated organs, including esophagus, eyes, lungs, tongue, bladder, and mucous membranes
- Headaches
- Stomach ulcers
- Appetite loss
- Coughing

Ask Jason to name the worst side effect from treatment, and he replies, "Just being sick, because you can't do anything. You have to stay in bed all day. Although," he adds brightly, "I got to know every star on the soap opera 'The Days of Our Lives.' "

Craig and I have yet to determine the long-term damage from *that*.

CHEMOTHERAPY DRUGS FOR PEDIATRIC CANCERS AND THEIR POTENTIAL SIDE EFFECTS

Asparaginase (also known as L-Asp, Amidohydrolase, Elspar)
Administered by injection to patients with acute leukemia

Side Effects Requiring Immediate Medical Attention:

- Labored breathing
- Joint pain
- Puffy face
- Skin rash or itching
- Stomach pain accompanied by severe nausea or vomiting

Side Effects Requiring Medical Attention as Soon as Possible:

- Jaundice
- Confusion, nervousness
- Drowsiness

CHEMOTHERAPY DRUGS FOR PEDIATRIC CANCERS AND THEIR POTENTIAL SIDE EFFECTS (cont.)

- Fever, chills, sore throat
- Pain in stomach or sides
- Hallucinations
- Depression
- Swollen feet or calves
- Lip and mouth sores
- Unusually frequent urination
- Extreme thirst
- Severe headaches
- Convulsions

Side Effects Generally Requiring No Medical Attention Unless Prolonged or Severe:

- Headache
- Appetite loss
- Nausea or vomiting
- Stomach cramps
- Weight loss

Bleomycin (also known as Blenoxane, BLM)
Administered by intravenous or intramuscular injection to patients with squamous-cell carcinoma, Hodgkin's disease, non-Hodgkin's lymphomas, testicular cancer

Side Effects Requiring Immediate Medical Attention:

- Fever and chills, usually occurring within three to six hours after dose
- Faintness, confusion
- Sweating
- Wheezing

Side Effects Requiring Medical Attention as Soon as Possible:

- Coughing
- Shortness of breath
- Mouth and lip sores

CHEMOTHERAPY DRUGS FOR PEDIATRIC CANCERS AND THEIR POTENTIAL SIDE EFFECTS (cont.)

Side Effects Generally Requiring No Medical Attention Unless Prolonged or Severe:

- Darkening or thickening of skin
- Itchy skin
- Rash or colored bumps on fingertips, elbows, or palms
- Red, tender skin
- Vomiting
- Appetite loss

Carmustine (also known as BCNU, BiCNU)
Administered by intravenous injection to patients with brain tumors, acute leukemia, Hodgkin's disease, non-Hodgkin's lymphomas

Side Effects Requiring Medical Attention as Soon as Possible:

- Coughing
- Fever, chills, sore throat
- Labored breathing
- Unusual bleeding or bruising
- Flushed face
- Mouth and lip sores
- Extreme fatigue or weakness
- Swollen feet or calves
- Decreased urination

Side Effects Generally Requiring No Medical Attention Unless Prolonged or Severe:

- Nausea or vomiting, usually lasting no longer than four to six hours
- Discolored skin along injected vein
- Diarrhea
- Difficulty swallowing
- Difficulty walking, dizziness
- Appetite loss
- Hair loss
- Skin rash, itchy skin

CHEMOTHERAPY DRUGS FOR PEDIATRIC CANCERS AND THEIR POTENTIAL SIDE EFFECTS (cont.)

Chlorambucil (also known as Leukeran)
Administered orally to patients with chronic leukemia, Hodgkin's disease, non-Hodgkin's lymphomas

Side Effects Requiring Medical Attention as Soon as Possible:

- Fever, chills, sore throat
- Mouth and lip sores
- Unusual bleeding or bruising
- Pain in stomach or sides
- Joint pain
- Skin rash
- Swollen feet or calves
- Convulsions
- Coughing
- Labored breathing
- Jaundice

Cisplatin (also known as Cisplatinum, Platinol, CDDP)
Administered by intravenous injection to patients with testicular cancer

Side Effects Requiring Immediate Medical Attention:

- Swollen face
- Heart palpitations
- Wheezing

Side Effects Requiring Medical Attention as Soon as Possible:

- Difficulty hearing, ringing in ears
- Fever, chills, sore throat
- Pain in stomach or sides
- Joint pain
- Swollen feet or calves
- Unusual bleeding or bruising

CHEMOTHERAPY DRUGS FOR PEDIATRIC CANCERS AND THEIR POTENTIAL SIDE EFFECTS (cont.)

- Loss of taste
- Extreme fatigue or weakness
- Numbness or tingling in fingers, toes, or face
- Blurry vision

Cyclophosphamide (also known as Cytoxan, Neosar)
Administered orally or by injection to patients with acute leukemia, Hodgkin's disease, non-Hodgkin's lymphomas, neuroblastoma, retino-blastoma

Side Effects Requiring Immediate Medical Attention:

- Bloody urine, painful urination
- Fever, chills, sore throat
- Unusual bleeding or bruising

Side Effects Requiring Medical Attention as Soon as Possible:

- Dizziness, confusion, or agitation
- In teenage girls, missed menstrual periods
- Fatigue
- Coughing
- Pain in stomach or sides
- Joint pain
- Labored breathing
- Swollen feet or calves
- Unusual bleeding or bruising
- Heart palpitations
- Black, tarry stools
- Mouth and lip sores
- Unusually frequent urination
- Jaundice

Side Effects Generally Requiring No Medical Attention Unless Prolonged or Severe:

CHEMOTHERAPY DRUGS FOR PEDIATRIC CANCERS AND THEIR POTENTIAL SIDE EFFECTS (cont.)

- Darkening of skin and fingernails
- Appetite loss
- Hair loss
- Nausea or vomiting

Cytarabine (also known as Ara-C, Cytosar-U, Cytosine, Arabinoside)
Administered by injection to patients with acute or chronic leukemia

Side Effects Requiring Medical Attention as Soon as Possible:

- Fever, chills, sore throat
- Unusual bleeding or bruising
- Pain in stomach or sides
- Joint pain
- Numbness or tingling in fingers, toes, or face
- Mouth and lip sores
- Swollen feet or calves
- Fatigue
- Black, tarry stools
- Bone or muscle pain
- Chest pain
- Coughing
- Difficulty swallowing
- Fainting spells
- General discomfort or weakness
- Heartburn
- Irregular heartbeat
- Pain at site of injection
- Reddened eyes
- Labored breathing
- Skin rash
- Decreased urination
- Jaundice

Side Effects Generally Requiring No Medical Attention Unless Prolonged or Severe:

CHEMOTHERAPY DRUGS FOR PEDIATRIC CANCERS
AND THEIR POTENTIAL SIDE EFFECTS (cont.)

- Appetite loss
- Nausea or vomiting

Dacarbazine (also known as DTIC-Dome)
Administered by intravenous injection to patients with Hodgkin's disease

Side Effects Requiring Medical Attention as Soon as Possible:

- Fever, chills, sore throat
- Unusual bleeding or bruising
- Mouth and lip sores

Side Effects Generally Requiring No Medical Attention Unless Prolonged or Severe:

- Appetite loss
- Nausea or vomiting, which should subside after one or two days

Dactinomycin (also known Cosmegen, Act-D, Actinomycin-D)
Administered by intravenous injection to patients with Wilms' tumor, rhabdomyosarcoma, bone sarcomas

Side Effects Requiring Immediate Medical Attention:

- Fever, chills, sore throat
- Unusual bleeding or bruising
- Wheezing

Side Effects Requiring Medical Attention as Soon as Possible:

- Black, tarry stools or chronic diarrhea
- Chronic stomach pain
- Difficulty swallowing
- Heartburn
- Mouth and lip sores

CHEMOTHERAPY DRUGS FOR PEDIATRIC CANCERS AND THEIR POTENTIAL SIDE EFFECTS (cont.)

- Joint pain
- Swollen feet or calves
- Jaundice

Side Effects Generally Requiring No Medical Attention Unless Prolonged or Severe:

- Darkened skin
- Hair loss
- Nausea or vomiting
- Reddened skin, skin rash or acne
- Fatigue

Daunorubicin (also known as Daunomycin, DMN, Cerubidine)
Administered by intravenous injection to patients with acute leukemia

Side Effects Requiring Immediate Medical Attention:

- Heart palpitations
- Pain at site of injection
- Labored breathing
- Swollen feet or calves
- Wheezing

Side Effects Requiring Medical Attention as Soon as Possible:

- Fever, chills, sore throat
- Mouth and lip sores
- Pain in stomach or sides
- Joint pain
- Unusual bleeding or bruising
- Skin rash, itchy skin

Side Effects Generally Requiring No Medical Attention Unless Prolonged or Severe:

CHEMOTHERAPY DRUGS FOR PEDIATRIC CANCERS AND THEIR POTENTIAL SIDE EFFECTS (cont.)

- Reddish urine, for one to two days after dose
- Hair loss
- Nausea or vomiting
- Darkened or reddened skin
- Diarrhea

Other Potential Side Effects:

- Heart damage, occurring most often in children under two

Dexamethasone (also known as Hexadrol, Decadron)
Administered orally or by intravenous injection to patients with acute leukemia, brain tumors

Side Effects Requiring Medical Attention as Soon as Possible:

- Impaired vision
- Weight gain, round face
- Suppression of fever or other signs of infection or inflammation
- Emotional changes
- Elevated blood pressure
- Increased thirst
- Increased urination
- Elevated blood sugar
- Hallucinations
- Skin rash, hives, acne
- Abdominal or stomach pain
- Bloody or black, tarry stools
- Hip pain
- Irregular heartbeat
- In teenage girls, menstrual problems
- Muscles cramps, pain, or weakness
- Nausea or vomiting
- Pain in back, ribs, arms, or legs
- Pitting or depression of skin at injection site
- Swollen feet or calves

CHEMOTHERAPY DRUGS FOR PEDIATRIC CANCERS AND THEIR POTENTIAL SIDE EFFECTS (cont.)

- Thin, "shiny" skin
- Unusual bruising
- Wounds that won't heal

Side Effects Generally Requiring No Medical Attention Unless Prolonged or Severe:

- Increased appetite
- False sense of well-being
- Nervousness, restlessness
- Difficulty sleeping
- Indigestion
- Darkening or lightening of skin color
- Headaches
- Unusual increase in hair growth on body or face
- Increased joint pain after injection into a joint

Doxorubicin (also known as Adriamycin)
Administered by intravenous injection to patients with acute leukemia, Wilms' tumor, neuroblastoma, soft-tissue sarcomas, bone sarcomas, Hodgkin's disease, non-Hodgkin's lymphomas, brain tumors

Side Effects Requiring Immediate Medical Attention:

- Heart palpitations
- Pain at site of injection
- Labored breathing
- Swollen feet or calves
- Wheezing

Side Effects Requiring Medical Attention as Soon as Possible:

- Fever, chills, sore throat
- Mouth and lip sores
- Pain in stomach or sides
- Joint pain

CHEMOTHERAPY DRUGS FOR PEDIATRIC CANCERS AND THEIR POTENTIAL SIDE EFFECTS (cont.)

- Unusual bleeding or bruising
- Skin rash, itchy skin

Side Effects Generally Requiring No Medical Attention Unless Prolonged or Severe:

- Hair loss
- Nausea or vomiting
- Reddish urine, for one to two days after dose
- Darkened soles, palms, or nails

Other Potential Side Effects:

- Heart damage, occurring most often in children under two

Etoposide (also known as VePesid and VP-16)
Administered by injection to patients with testicular cancer

Side Effects Requiring Medical Attention as Soon as Possible:

- Fever, chills, sore throat
- Mouth and lip sores
- Unusual bleeding or bruising
- Difficulty walking
- Numbness or tingling in fingers and toes
- Pain at site of injection
- Labored breathing
- Weakness

Side Effects Generally Requiring No Medical Attention Unless Prolonged or Severe:

- Appetite loss
- Hair loss
- Nausea or vomiting

CHEMOTHERAPY DRUGS FOR PEDIATRIC CANCERS AND THEIR POTENTIAL SIDE EFFECTS (cont.)

- Diarrhea
- Extreme fatigue

Fluorouracil (also known as 5-FU, Adrucil)
Administered by injection to patients with colon cancer, stomach cancer, pancreatic cancer, and other extremely rare pediatric malignancies

Side Effects Requiring Immediate Medical Attention:

- Diarrhea or black, tarry stools
- Fever, chills, sore throat
- Heartburn
- Severe nausea or vomiting
- Stomach cramps
- Unusual bleeding or bruising

Side Effects Requiring Medical Attention as Soon as Possible:

- Chest pain
- Coughing
- Lack of balance
- Labored breathing

Side Effects Generally Requiring No Medical Attention Unless Prolonged or Severe:

- Appetite loss
- Hair loss
- Skin rash, itchy skin
- Nausea or vomiting
- Weakness

Hydrocortisone (also known as Hydrocortone, Solu-cortef)
Administered by intravenous injection or orally to patients with acute leukemia

CHEMOTHERAPY DRUGS FOR PEDIATRIC CANCERS AND THEIR POTENTIAL SIDE EFFECTS (cont.)

Side Effects Requiring Medical Attention as Soon as Possible:

- Impaired vision
- Weight gain, round face
- Suppression of fever or other signs of infection or inflammation
- Emotional changes
- Elevated blood pressure
- Increased thirst
- Increased urination
- Elevated blood sugar
- Hallucinations
- Skin rash, hives, acne
- Abdominal or stomach pain
- Bloody or black, tarry stools
- Hip pain
- Irregular heartbeat
- In teenage girls, menstrual problems
- Muscles cramps, pain, or weakness
- Nausea or vomiting
- Pain in back, ribs, arms, or legs
- Pitting or depression of skin at injection site
- Swollen feet or calves
- Thin, "shiny" skin
- Unusual bruising
- Wounds that won't heal

Side Effects Generally Requiring No Medical Attention Unless Prolonged or Severe:

- Increased appetite
- False sense of well-being
- Nervousness, restlessness
- Difficulty sleeping
- Indigestion
- Darkening or lightening of skin color
- Headaches

CHEMOTHERAPY DRUGS FOR PEDIATRIC CANCERS AND THEIR POTENTIAL SIDE EFFECTS (cont.)

- Unusual increase in hair growth on body or face
- Increased joint pain after injection into a joint

Hydroxyurea (also known as Hydrea)
Administered orally to patients with chronic leukemia, melanoma, squamous-cell carcinoma

Side Effects Requiring Medical Attention as Soon as Possible:

- Fever, chills, sore throat
- Mouth and lip sores
- Unusual bleeding or bruising
- Convulsions
- Dizziness, confusion
- Hallucinations
- Pain in stomach or sides
- Joint pain
- Swollen feet or calves

Side Effects Generally Requiring No Medical Attention Unless Prolonged or Severe:

- Diarrhea
- Drowsiness
- Appetite loss
- Nausea or vomiting

Lomustine (also known as CCNU and CeeNu)
Administered orally to patients with brain tumors, Hodgkin's disease

Side Effects Requiring Medical Attention as Soon as Possible:

- Fever, chills, sore throat
- Unusual bleeding or bruising
- Awkwardness, confusion
- Slurred speech

CHEMOTHERAPY DRUGS FOR PEDIATRIC CANCERS AND THEIR POTENTIAL SIDE EFFECTS (cont.)

- Mouth and lip sores
- Swollen feet or calves
- Decreased urination
- Extreme fatigue, weakness
- Jaundice
- Coughing
- Labored breathing

Side Effects Generally Requiring No Medical Attention Unless Prolonged or Severe:

- Appetite loss
- Nausea or vomiting, usually up to twenty-four hours after dose
- Darkened skin
- Diarrhea
- Hair loss
- Skin rash, itchy skin

Mechlorethamine (also known as Mustargen, Nitrogen Mustard) Administered by intravenous injection to patients with chronic leukemia, Hodgkin's disease, mycosis fungoides (skin lymphoma)

Side Effects Requiring Immediate Medical Attention:

- Wheezing

Side Effects Requiring Medical Attention as Soon as Possible:

- Fever, chills, sore throat
- In teenage girls, missed menstrual periods
- Painful rash
- Unusual bleeding or bruising
- Dizziness
- Pain in stomach and sides
- Hearing loss, ringing in ears

CHEMOTHERAPY DRUGS FOR PEDIATRIC CANCERS AND THEIR POTENTIAL SIDE EFFECTS (cont.)

- Swollen feet or calves
- Numbness, tingling, or burning of fingers, toes, or face
- Jaundice

Side Effects Generally Requiring No Medical Attention Unless Prolonged or Severe:

- Nausea or vomiting, usually lasting between eight and twenty-four hours

Mercaptopurine (also known as Purinethol)
Administered orally to patients with acute leukemia, central-nervous-system leukemia

Side Effects Requiring Medical Attention as Soon as Possible:

- Fever, chills, sore throat
- Unusual bleeding or bruising
- Extreme fatigue, weakness
- Jaundice
- Appetite loss
- Pain in stomach or sides
- Joint pain
- Nausea or vomiting
- Swollen feet or calves
- Black, tarry stools
- Mouth and lip sores

Methotrexate (also known as Mexate, MTX, Folex)
Administered orally or by injection to patients with acute leukemia, non-Hodgkin's lymphomas, bone sarcomas

Side Effects Requiring Immediate Medical Attention:

CHEMOTHERAPY DRUGS FOR PEDIATRIC CANCERS AND THEIR POTENTIAL SIDE EFFECTS (cont.)

- Black, tarry stools, or diarrhea
- Bloody vomit
- Stomach pain
- Mouth and lip sores

Side Effects Requiring Medical Attention as Soon as Possible:

- Fever, chills, sore throat
- Unusual bleeding or bruising
- Bloody or dark urine
- Blurred vision
- Confusion, dizziness
- Convulsions or seizures
- Coughing
- Fatigue, extreme weakness
- Headaches
- Joint pain
- Labored breathing
- Swollen feet or calves
- Jaundice

Side Effects Generally Requiring No Medical Attention Unless Prolonged or Severe:

- Appetite loss
- Nausea or vomiting

Other Potential Side Effects:

- Extreme sensitivity to sunlight; avoid too much sun, and call your child's doctor immediately in the event of a severe burn

Plicamycin (also known as Mithracin, Mithramycin)
Administered by injection to patients with testicular cancer

Side Effects Requiring Immediate Medical Attention:

CHEMOTHERAPY DRUGS FOR PEDIATRIC CANCERS AND THEIR POTENTIAL SIDE EFFECTS (cont.)

- Bloody or black, tarry stools
- Flushed, red, or swollen face
- Skin rash or red-spotted skin
- Sore throat, fever
- Nosebleeds
- Unusual bleeding or bruising
- Bloody vomit

Side Effects Generally Requiring No Medical Attention Unless Prolonged or Severe:

- Diarrhea
- Irritated, sore mouth
- Appetite loss
- Nausea or vomiting
- Drowsiness
- Fever
- Headaches
- Depression
- Pain, redness or soreness at site of injection
- Extreme fatigue, weakness

Prednisone (also known as Deltasone, Meticorten, Orasone)
Administered orally to patients with acute leukemia, non-Hodgkin's lymphomas

Side Effects Requiring Medical Attention as Soon as Possible:

- Impaired, blurry vision; seeing "halos" around lights
- Frequent urination
- Extreme thirst
- Skin rash, acne, or other skin problems
- Back or rib pain
- Bloody or black, tarry stools
- Round face
- Irregular heartbeats

CHEMOTHERAPY DRUGS FOR PEDIATRIC CANCERS AND THEIR POTENTIAL SIDE EFFECTS (cont.)

- In teenage girls, menstrual problems
- Depression, mood changes
- Muscle cramps, pain, weakness
- Nausea or vomiting
- Sore throat, fever
- Stomach pain or burning
- Swollen feet or calves
- Extreme fatigue, weakness
- Wounds that won't heal

Side Effects Generally Requiring No Medical Attention Unless Prolonged or Severe:

- Indigestion
- False sense of well-being
- Increased appetite
- Nervousness, restlessness
- Trouble sleeping
- Weight gain

Procarbazine (also known as Matulane and Natulan)
Administered orally to patients with Hodgkin's disease

Side Effects Requiring Immediate Medical Attention:

- Severe headaches
- Stiff neck
- Heart palpitations
- Nausea or vomiting

Side Effects Requiring Medical Attention as Soon as Possible:

- Black, tarry stools or diarrhea
- Convulsions
- Bloody vomit
- Coughing

CHEMOTHERAPY DRUGS FOR PEDIATRIC CANCERS AND THEIR POTENTIAL SIDE EFFECTS (cont.)

- Fever, chills, sore throat
- Hallucinations
- In teenage girls, missed menstrual periods
- Labored breathing
- Thickening of bronchial secretions
- Extreme fatigue, weakness
- Unusual bleeding or bruising
- Mouth and lip sores
- Tingling or numbness of fingers or toes
- Unsteadiness, awkwardness
- Jaundice
- Fainting
- Skin rash or hives, itchy skin
- Wheezing

Side Effects Generally Requiring No Medical Attention Unless Prolonged or Severe:

- Drowsiness
- Muscle or joint pain
- Muscle twitching
- Nervousness
- Sleeplessness, nightmares
- Nausea or vomiting
- Sweating
- Extreme fatigue, weakness
- Darkened skin
- Dizziness or light-headedness when getting up from a reclining or sitting position
- Flushed face

Thioguanine (also known as 6-TG)
Administered orally to patients with acute leukemia

Side Effects Requiring Immediate Medical Attention:

CHEMOTHERAPY DRUGS FOR PEDIATRIC CANCERS
AND THEIR POTENTIAL SIDE EFFECTS (cont.)

- Fever, chills, sore throat
- Unusual bleeding or bruising

Side Effects Requiring Medical Attention as Soon as Possible:

- Pain in stomach or sides
- Joint pain
- Swollen feet or calves
- Difficulty walking
- Jaundice
- Black, tarry stools
- Mouth and lip sores

Side Effects Generally Requiring No Medical Attention Unless Prolonged or Severe:

- Nausea or vomiting
- Appetite loss
- Diarrhea
- Skin rash, itchy skin

Vinblastine (also known as Velban, VLB)
Administered by intravenous injection to patients with Hodgkin's disease, non-Hodgkin's lymphomas, testicular cancer

Side Effects Requiring Medical Attention as Soon as Possible:

- Fever, chills, sore throat
- Pain in stomach or sides
- Swollen feet or calves
- Unusual bleeding or bruising
- Black, tarry stools
- Difficulty walking
- Double vision, drooping eyelids
- Headaches
- Jaw pain

CHEMOTHERAPY DRUGS FOR PEDIATRIC CANCERS AND THEIR POTENTIAL SIDE EFFECTS (cont.)

- Depression
- Numbness, tingling, or pain in fingers and toes
- Pain in boys' testicles
- Mouth and lip sores
- Extreme weakness

Side Effects Generally Requiring No Medical Attention Unless Prolonged or Severe:

- Hair loss
- Muscle pain
- Nausea or vomiting

Vincristine (also known as Oncovin, VCR)
Administered by intravenous injection to patients with Hodgkin's disease, non-Hodgkin's lymphomas, rhabdomyosarcoma, neuroblastoma, Wilms' tumor

Side Effects Requiring Medical Attention as Soon as Possible:

- Blurred or double vision, drooping eyelids
- Constipation
- Difficulty walking
- Pain in stomach or sides
- Headaches
- Jaw pain
- Joint pain
- Numbness, tingling, or pain in fingers and toes
- Pain in boys' testicles
- Swollen feet or calves
- Extreme weakness
- Agitation
- Bed-wetting
- Confusion
- Dizziness or light-headedness when getting up from a reclining or sitting position

CHEMOTHERAPY DRUGS FOR PEDIATRIC CANCERS AND THEIR POTENTIAL SIDE EFFECTS (cont.)

- Convulsions, seizures
- Hallucinations
- Lack of sweating
- Appetite loss
- Depression
- Painful or difficult urination, decreased or increased urination
- Difficulty sleeping
- Unconsciousness
- Coughing
- Fever, chills, sore throat
- Labored breathing
- Mouth and lip sores
- Unusual bleeding or bruising

Side Effects Generally Requiring No Medical Attention Unless Prolonged or Severe:

- Hair loss
- Bloating
- Diarrhea
- Weight loss
- Nausea or vomiting
- Skin rash

Adapted from "Chemotherapy & You/A Guide to Self-Help During Treatment" (1987) and "Young People With Cancer/A Handbook for Parents" (1989), both published by the U.S. Department of Health and Human Services; *USP DI, Volume II, Advice for the Patient,* copyright, the United States Pharmacopeial Convention, Inc., permission granted; *1991 Physicians' Desk Reference,* published by Medical Economics Data, Oradell, New Jersey; and *Handbook of Pediatric Oncology* (1989), published by Little, Brown and Company, Boston, Massachusetts.

CHAPTER SIX

PARTICIPATING IN YOUR CHILD'S TREATMENT

Typical Childrens' Anxieties • Comforting Young
Patients • Assisting the Medical Staff • Low-Cost Lodging

Unless someone close to us has suffered a serious illness, our perceptions about sickness are formed mainly from novels, movies, and television. The prevailing portrayal casts patients as heroes and heroines who respond bravely in their time of crisis. Perhaps we cling to that image because all of us, the ill and loved ones alike, need to believe in it. But based on our experiences with Jason, my father, and other relatives who've wrestled with life-threatening maladies, I'd suggest that people simply behave in character. The stress and uncertainty merely exaggerate the personality you already know.

However, sometimes adversity brings out a person's exceptional qualities. Certainly that was true of Jason. From the moment of diagnosis our six-year-old displayed remarkable courage. When faced with painful tests and treatments, often he was the one who said optimistically, "Come on, Mom, we can do this."

"Jake went through it all a lot better than his dad did," Craig says today. Yet if you had asked us beforehand which son would be least equipped to cope with pediatric cancer, we'd have said Jason. Of the three boys he seemed the most vulnerable: quiet and shy, a bit standoffish around other children. While Tim sailed through first grade, his twin struggled somewhat. "Jason was always different," my husband contends, "even as a baby."

Looking back, I see that Jason wasn't defenseless, possessing all along an inner strength many adults would envy. I don't believe he changed as a result of his illness, it just took his having cancer to reveal that side of him to us.

In this chapter we will examine the typical emotions, anxieties, and fears that beset young patients. All parents in this situation feel frustrated by their powerlessness to help their child. The outcome, after all, rests primarily in the hands of the medical staff and may even be beyond their control. But as you will see, there are many ways to comfort children and to participate actively in their treatment. In helping your child you'll also be helping yourself.

TYPICAL CHILDREN'S ANXIETIES

Fear of Separation from Parents

Hospitalized youngsters under age five often feel abandoned, lonely, and frightened. Anytime you leave them, they may need reassurance that you will come back. During Jason's stay in Saint Marys, he didn't want me to go, so I camped out there day and night. Given everything he'd been through, who could blame him?

After a few days of not eating regularly, I started losing weight, which concerned a visiting uncle of mine. "You need to get some food in you," he said.

"Oh, no," I replied, shaking my head, "I can't leave my son." Had Uncle Francis not insisted, I probably would have anchored myself at Jason's bedside.

My uncle quietly explained to him, "We spoke to the nurse, and she said you won't be having any tests for a couple of hours. So I'm going to take your mother to a restaurant just across the street. Your grandma will be here with you, and we'll be back real soon."

"Okay," said Jason. *Like, no problem.*

I've seen parents enlist a nurse to distract their youngster as they slip out the door. It seems to me that sneaking away would only exacerbate a child's anxiety. Usually kids can be calmed through verbal assurances that nothing painful or upsetting will take place while Mom or Dad is gone. The nursing staff can consult your child's chart to inform you of upcoming in-room medications, examinations, blood tests—anything that might distress her. Then plan your absences accordingly.

Other than that one brief excursion I never left Jason's room. I realize this may not be possible for all parents, particularly single or working mothers and fathers. In the event that you can't be with your child, arrange for a friend or family member to visit. But there are certain times when it's essential that parents be present:

• During all crucial tests and procedures
• Before and after surgery
• The patient's first night of hospitalization

As we noted in Chapter Three, many hospitals have relaxed restrictions on parental visiting, and the more accommodating facilities provide beds for parents either in the patient's room or somewhere on the same floor. At the very least you should be permitted to snooze in a chair in the room.

It's vital to your child's welfare that she never feel alone, especially during times of stress. A recent study disclosed that hospitalized youngsters whose parents visited regularly recovered faster than those whose parents did not. Furthermore anxious children may revert to bedwetting, thumb sucking, baby talk, and other regressive behavior.

Fear of Mutilation, Bodily Harm

Kids between ages six and ten frequently worry more about losing a limb to cancer than about dying. Ever since the publication of Jason's *My Book for Kids with Cansur,* young patients have called our son to confide their concerns, chief of which is the prospect of mutilation. "Are the doctors going to cut off my leg?" these children want to know, responding just as Jason did upon learning he had cancer.

Despite repeated assurances, my six-year-old felt the need to bring up the matter every so often. Each time, I explained that in all likelihood he wouldn't lose an arm or a leg "because the cancer's not in your bones, honey."

Jason also fields calls from children who do face amputation, one of them a twelve-year-old scheduled for surgery the next day. "Did you ever see a kid with his leg cut off?" he asked. My son told him about Jim, a counselor we met during a visit to a Michigan camp for kids with cancer. The athletic young man lugged our baggage from the airplane to the car, escorted us to the camp, and worked up a sweat shooting baskets with Jason all day. It wasn't until bedtime that we discovered Jim had a prosthetic leg, due to osteosarcoma.

"Your life isn't over just because you don't have a leg," Jason consoled the nervous twelve-year-old. "Plenty of people with artificial legs get to do lots of neat things and live normally."

Self-Pity, Resentment, Anger

What cancer patient hasn't felt sorry for himself at one time or another? "The first time I had chemotherapy," says Jason, "I thought, *What did I do to deserve this?*" Every now and then he grumbled, "This stinks!" or "Why does this have to happen to me?" Certainly patients are entitled to a degree of self-pity. But our son never wallowed in it. If he had, Craig and I wouldn't have let him for long. That destructive emotion only contributes to feelings of hopelessness, which can actually depress the body's immune system.

Teenagers, even when healthy, seem to resist authority *just because.* Some teen patients lash out at the medical staff, which in their eyes has replaced the disease itself as the villain. They fuss and fidget during tests, suddenly develop lockjaw when it's time to swallow medicine, and in general refuse to cooperate.

Younger kids may reject their parents for "letting" them get sick, hissing, "I hate you!" or "Go away, leave me alone!" The pain of treatment shatters their faith in Mom and Dad as their protectors. One of the most heartbreaking scenes Craig and I witnessed was a seriously ill eight-year-old boy in the Saint Marys intensive-care ward. Over and over he hollered, "I'm gonna die! I'm gonna die!" You just wanted to wrap your arms around the poor child. But he wouldn't let his mother or father hold him. Whenever anyone came near him, he shrieked, "Don't touch me! Get away from me! Don't touch me!"

Though I never got to know his folks, I can imagine their anguish. Parents in this circumstance must remember that in spite of their child's resentment, he still loves them. Unable to direct his anger at the cancer, and perhaps aware of his dependence on the doctors and nurses, he vents it on them instead.

It is believed that these outbursts may also be a way for a youngster to *protect* her parents, by pushing them away. In the child's subconscious mind the alienating behavior will make it so that Mom and Dad won't miss her as much after she's gone. For a similar reason some kids withdraw emotionally. The National Cancer Institute advises that a member of the health-care team not directly involved with treatment can often succeed at drawing out a hostile or incommunicative patient.

Still other children's targets are more random. One mother we met was sick with worry over her seven-year-old son, a churning volcano of bitterness. When told that he would have to return to the Mayo Clinic for observation due to a high fever, the boy stalked into the garage and stomped to death a litter of newborn kittens. "He has this rage bubbling inside him," the woman lamented.

To be sure, Jason wasn't always an angel. Some days it was a struggle to get him to take his antinausea medicine, which he'd dump in the wastebasket. Other days he simply bit the bullet, growling, "Give it here," then tossing back the Phenergan and Benadryl with a grimace. Fortunately, when it came to acting grumpy, the two of us usually managed to work alternate shifts. The times Jason misbehaved, I happened to have a surplus of patience. And the times my nerves jangled, he was chipper.

Dr. Bringelsen characterizes Jason as "full of spunk and feisty." In short a typical young patient. "He fought like a tiger sometimes," she says, adding with a laugh, "He didn't write about *that* in his book. Jason never refused to do anything we asked him, he just let us know he didn't always like it, which is fine. That's a lot healthier than a passive kid."

Physicians and nurses actually worry more about overly submissive, apathetic children, for a combative spirit and a will to survive are critical to overcoming any serious illness. Youngsters who act out their emotions and relieve tension tend to feel less anxious than those who internalize it. The dilemma confronting parents of the latter child is how to heal wounds that are concealed.

ENCOURAGE CHILDREN TO
TALK ABOUT THEIR CANCER

Most kids need to discuss their condition, though they may not always volunteer to do so. When do you know whether or not to prod? Your child will give you the signal. Jason, an unusually expressive little boy, frequently raised the subject in the evening. We'd be lying on the couch together, my son dressed for bed in his pajamas, when suddenly he'd pipe up, "Harlan's going to die, isn't he?"

"Well, maybe, yes."

"I wonder if he's scared." We'd talk about it until Jason seemed satisfied.

Many times I flubbed my cue, thinking he needed to talk when in fact cancer was the last thing he wanted to think about. If he seemed bummed out about something, I might ask, "What's the matter?" to which Jason might snap, *"Nothin'."* Whoa. End of conversation.

Mothers and fathers will sometimes avoid the issue entirely for fear of saying the "wrong thing." I believe patients and parents benefit from any heartfelt discussion. But communicating, listening, and tending to an ill youngster's emotional needs are *skills* that for most of us require practice. Some guidelines to follow are:

- Don't dictate how he "should" feel or tell him, "I understand exactly what you're going through." You don't, and by defining his feelings you appear not to be truly listening to him.
- Don't pressure him into pretending he feels fine because it's what you want to hear.
- Don't fudge an answer to a treatment-related question when you really don't know. Tell your child you'll ask his doctor and find out.
- Don't discourage talk you consider morbid, for example about amputation or death. Patients need to openly discuss with their parents anything weighing on their minds.
- Don't minimize the gravity of their condition. Instead of a patronizing (and unconvincing) "Don't worry, everything will be fine," say, "This treatment may be tough, but if we do what we're supposed to, I believe you'll be okay."
- Don't let your child blame himself for his illness. This is an all-too-

common reaction among kids, who guiltily believe they somehow brought about their cancer through past misdeeds. Besides reassuring him he's done nothing wrong, stress that disease isn't a form of punishment meted out by whichever higher power you worship.

- *Do* ask questions: "What are you thinking?" "How do you feel about what the doctor said?" Encourage your child to express his fears, and then *listen.*
- *Do* explain that it's all right to feel sad, depressed, or to cry; that bottling up emotions isn't healthy.
- *Do* engage your child in conversations about topics other than his health, whether it be sports, music, school, or plain old gossip. Kids stricken with a serious illness feel isolated enough. It's important to keep them plugged into the world beyond their hospital room.
- *Do* sympathize with a patient who is feeling down. But try gently to guide the conversation in a more positive direction.
- *Do* train yourself to read between the lines by becoming an active listener. Many youngsters either deny, are numb to, or simply cannot articulate their true feelings. One way to help a child acknowledge how he really feels is to repeat his thoughts back to him, underscoring the vital points. For instance, he might express deep concern about who may be sleeping in his room at home or sitting at his desk in school. What he's really worried about is being replaced and forgotten.
- *Do* remind him that he is not alone in his fight. Shower him with unconditional love and support. The recuperative effect of a parent's "I love you" cannot be underestimated.

As for inadvertently upsetting a child by divulging the severity of his illness, the same information that frightens one child empowers another. You have to gauge carefully how much your youngster probably wants to hear, following Chapter One's age guidelines for breaking the news of a cancer diagnosis. It bears repeating, though, that patients kept unaware may imagine things far worse than they really are. Craig and I found that so long as we conveyed hope, we could talk to our son frankly without dampening his spirits.

A good way to get children to open up is for patients and parents to read about pediatric cancer, either together or separately, and then discuss the material. This is how Jason came to write his own book, by

my reading to him. Below we've recommended free booklets and coloring books that, in addition to being informative, contain the reflections
of other kids with cancer. Your child will surely appreciate and relate
to their often touching anecdotes about what it's like to have cancer.

From the National Cancer Institute (800-4-CANCER):

• "Help Yourself: Tips for Teenagers with Cancer"
• "Hospital Days/Treatment Ways Coloring Book"

From the American Cancer Society (regional offices, 800-ACS-2345;
national office, 404-320-3333):

• "What Happened to You Happened to Me"

From the Leukemia Society of America (chapters are located in fifty-six
cities nationwide—check your local white pages or call the toll-free LSA
information hotline at 800-955-4LSA; national office, 212-573-8484):

• "Learn About Leukemia: A Coloring and Activity Book"
• "What Is It That I Have, Don't Want, Didn't Ask For, Can't Give
  Back, and How I Feel About It"

A PARENT'S COMFORTING PRESENCE

Jason says the best part of being hospitalized, if there is such a thing,
was his dad's stories. Craig kept our six-year-old transfixed with tall
tales about the stuffed animals in the Saint Marys activity room, who
kept him company at night.

"Boy, Jake," he'd begin, "you ought to sleep in there sometime,
because after everyone goes to bed, those animals talk. I could hardly
get any sleep. The elephant and the lion, they go on about the dumbest
stuff. . . ." Of course Jason ate this right up. *"Really? They said that?"*
The stories grew so popular that pretty soon kids on the floor flocked
into Jason's room to hear about the chatty stuffed critters down the hall.

Sometimes the most comforting sound from a child's hospital room, though, is the silence of parent and patient absorbed in their own activities. At first you feel compelled perpetually to entertain your youngster, when in fact your mere presence is usually comforting enough. Jason liked for me to lie next to him in bed, but didn't always need for us to do something together. While I watched TV, he might quietly color or play with his Superman figures, perfectly satisfied. On nights when he felt restless, I lightly massaged his scalp, which helped him to relax and drift off to sleep.

GIVING PATIENTS CHOICES

Perhaps the cruelest consequence pediatric cancer inflicts on children isn't so much the deprivation of health but of control—over their bodies, their daily lives, their futures. Teenagers find these losses especially frustrating. Therefore doctors, nurses, and parents should make every effort to permit patients some say in their therapy, as long as their health isn't jeopardized.

Involving kids in treatment by giving them choices restores a measure of control, albeit limited, against their disease. Granted, the options boil down to seemingly insignificant matters such as choosing which flavor juice to drink with oral medicine. But to kids stripped of their autonomy, merely picking orange over grape lets them feel they can help themselves.

"There's no question that patients who are actively involved feel better sooner," Dr. Smithson contends. "We often say that patients do better with any problem they focus on and work on.

"It won't cure cancer," he emphasizes, "and there are some things that are going to take their own course of time for recovery no matter what. But it does help overall to enhance the process and probably gives patients the strength to do what's necessary to get the cancer under control."

Decisions that can be deferred to children include:

• Selecting veins for I.V. insertions
• Whether to apply rubbing alcohol themselves prior to I.V.'s or injections, or to have a nurse do it
• Whose hand to hold

- The order of injections
- Their bath time
- Scheduling doctors' appointments themselves

Says Dr. Bringelsen, "We try to give young patients as much leeway as we can," to make them feel more like participants than victims. Hospitalized youngsters are encouraged to wear their own clothes, keep themselves groomed, exercise (even if it means just roaming the halls, I.V. poles in tow), entertain friends, and eat meals in the cafeteria, provided they feel up to it.

Approximately 80 percent of U.S. medical facilities run what are called Child Life programs, designed to further uplift kids' spirits. At Saint Marys the staff regularly threw pizza parties complete with balloons and hats for kids finishing treatment. What a delight it was to hear laughter echo through the hallways.

Next to Jason's room sat the activity room, a spacious, sunny, comfortably furnished area bulging with books, magazines, games, musical instruments, dolls, toys, and of course Craig's stuffed nighttime companions. Other hospitals' recreation areas stock favorite amusements such as video games, videocassette recorders, and audio equipment.

Playtime isn't just for diverting kids from the trauma and interminable boredom of hospital stays, but has evolved into an essential element of therapy. Through observing the children at play and talking with them, Child Life workers, social workers, recreational therapists, psychologists, and similar professionals help youngsters surmount their fears.

At one end of the room stood a mock treatment center where kids could play doctor, sticking teddy bears with play needles and administering "I.V.'s" to plastic dolls. The idea is to make the procedures less intimidating. In the hobby area, meanwhile, budding Picassos at easels painted their anxieties. A child's depiction of her parents as monsters, for example, would reveal to a recreational therapist that she felt angry with them for "subjecting" her to pain.

Child Life workers visit bedridden youngsters in their rooms, which can be personalized with reminders from home. Bring favorite blankets, toys, and clothing, familiar items that your child can focus on. "I brought a poster and hung it above my bed," remembers Jason. "It said, 'Help Me to Remember, Lord, That Nothing's Going to Happen Today That You and I Can't Handle Together.'

"And whenever I felt scared, I kneeled on my bed and read it."

PARENTS PARTICIPATING IN THERAPY

Parents, as well as children, need to take an active role in their treatment. Seeing Craig and me cooperating with the medical team inspired Jason's greater trust in them.

Nurses' responsibilities have continually expanded to encompass duties once overseen exclusively by physicians. I worked closely with Donna Betcher, a nurse-practitioner and clinical-nurse specialist of pediatric oncology. Warm, outgoing, with an open, friendly face, she'd been at the Mayo Clinic since 1972. Jason thought Donna was the greatest.

Still, he preferred that I tend to as many of his personal needs as possible. Though only six, he felt self-conscious about strangers giving him sponge baths, enemas, and so on. When hospitalized a second time, in September, he'd lost so much weight that he developed sore joints from lying in bed. The nurses used to vigorously rub him all over with lotion to stimulate the circulation. "My mom can do that," Jason told them. "Just give her the cream." Without a word of objection they handed me the bottle, briefly instructed me on what to do, and left the room.

The entire staff encouraged me to perform whatever routine tasks I could, from emptying bedpans to gripping my son's hand during blood tests. Some medical centers even allow parents in the operating room to comfort their child while anesthesia is administered. Depending on your hospital's regulations, other ways to assist a young patient include:

• Taking his temperature and blood pressure
• Changing dressings
• Giving back rubs
• Bathing him in bed or assisting him during showers
• Seeing that he shifts positions in bed, to prevent bedsores
• Informing the medical staff of the child's likes and dislikes

Today's pediatric-oncology nurses care for youngsters in so many ways, there's always the occasional parent who feels displaced. As Nurse Betcher acknowledges, "One issue that comes up repeatedly is parents claiming the nursing staff sometimes spoils the kids, let's say by failing to impose the same restrictions they would. But then, sometimes we have to set restrictions at the clinic that parents have trouble enforcing at home, which also might be hard for the parent." I can honestly say those thoughts never entered my mind. On the contrary I felt forever grateful to the nurses for their diligence and expertise.

No matter how conscientious the staff, foul-ups and oversights concerning treatment inevitably occur. A parent's prime responsibility toward a young patient is to act as her advocate and speak up for her when necessary. For example, because resident doctors and nurses rotate approximately every four weeks, it's conceivable that parents might come to know their child's drug schedule and dosages better than someone brand-new to her case.

Should you suspect a doctor or nurse of preparing an incorrect or unscheduled medication, insist that one of the attending physicians or the chief of service double-check it. According to one study, 50 percent of parents surveyed claimed they'd had to intervene to prevent medical mistakes. In addition to improper dosages, the situations most often cited involved radiation procedures, rapport between children and staff, continuity of care, and I.V. insertions. Regarding the latter, you'll remember my husband's once having to stop a student doctor from using Jason's hand as a pincushion.

Keep a Journal

Before our brief return home at the beginning of July, Dr. Burgert had sketched for me the chemotherapy's potential side effects. "When you bring Jason back in seven days," he said, "if he has a bruise on his leg and I ask you, 'Where did he get this?' I want you to be able to tell me, 'He got it playing baseball Monday afternoon around two o'clock, and by Wednesday it was blue.'

"I want you to have specifics," the doctor explained, "so if you need to, write them down."

From that day on I recorded in a daily journal anything I felt might be of value to Jason's physicians, beginning with the dates and results of my son's first blood tests. I don't know if Dr. Burgert suggested that every parent keep a log, or if he just intuited that I needed to maintain some control, but the spiral appointment book quickly filled up with entries specifying:

• **Diagnostic Tests**—date, type, and location of test and results

• **Chemotherapy**—date and location of treatment; drug(s) given; method(s) of administration

• **Other Medications**—(vitamins, antacids, pain relievers, and so on)—date given; dose and frequency; name of prescribing or recommending doctor.

• **Radiation**—date and location of treatment; body site; type of radiation machine used; number of rads delivered

• **Pain and other side effects**—symptom; date first noticed; running commentary tracking its progression or regression; severity of pain, expressed in a number from one to ten and descriptive words such as "shooting," "numbing," or "throbbing"

• **Miscellaneous Information**—child's temperature, activity level, sleeping patterns, emotions

Some days my entries consisted of only a few words: "Good day. No problems." Other times I had so many notes and questions to jot down that my handwriting spilled over into the next date's space. I must confess that I probably went overboard, documenting every minute detail of Jason's life down to what he ate for each meal. *If he gets over this disease*, I thought, *maybe this information can be useful for cancer research.*

I'm not so sure I was wrong. Jason went two years without a blood transfusion, unusual for a child receiving such aggressive chemotherapy. Studying my journal, one of his physicians remarked, "This kid eats more oatmeal than anybody I've ever seen." Which was true. Jason wolfed it down for breakfast, after school, and before bedtime. The doctor speculated, "Maybe that's why Jason's blood is so rich in iron and builds back up so fast."

Dr. Bringelsen says, "Being able to refer to Geralyn's notes was invaluable, and I think it helped her a lot too. We encourage parents to keep journals. For instance if one antinausea medicine proves to be especially effective, the parents can jot that down and tell the doctor the next time, 'Try that again; it really worked well.'

"It's helpful to have that sort of written information, because our medical records aren't always so detailed. We know *what* we gave, but we might not know how well it worked for that particular child."

PREPARING A CHILD FOR PAIN

The prospect of pain provokes considerable anxiety among young patients, especially before new treatments. "One of the most important things parents can do," contends Dr. Bringelsen, "is to be very honest with their child: acknowledge that the procedures are hard and may hurt, but at the same time support the medical staff who have to do these things." As Craig once told our son, "Sometimes the doctors are going to hurt you in order to make you better."

Jason is glad we chose to be upfront. "I wanted to know what to expect," he says. "It's a good thing my mom and dad were always straight with me, because if you can't trust your parents, you have no one to turn to. When they told me something didn't hurt, I didn't have to worry about it."

Nurse Betcher used to inform us a month ahead of time which tests were scheduled and how much discomfort to anticipate, but left it up to us when to tell Jason. "That's the best way," she says. "Some kids who know they're going to have a bone-marrow aspiration in two weeks will stew about it the entire time, while others will use those two weeks to prepare themselves mentally.

"It's very important, though, that children know whether or not they're going to undergo a procedure," she stresses. Parents who deceive their youngsters—claiming no tests are planned when they know for a fact they are—irreparably betray their children's trust.

Occasionally the night before or the day of a painful or unfamiliar procedure, Jason grew quiet, to this day a signal that he's nervous and upset. In a small voice he'd say, "Mom, I'm really scared about this one."

"Well, what are you nervous about, honey? You've been through this before." Together we'd rehearse the treatment aloud, step-by-step, speculating on the worst that could happen. Kids often find that discussing fears aloud or writing them down, rather than mulling them over silently, helps to overcome their fright.

Be conscious, however, of the language you use. It's easy to assume that your child understands, when in fact she's misinterpreted *dye* as *die*, causing needless worry. After describing upcoming treatments to Jason and explaining why they were necessary, I used to ask him to repeat in his own words what I'd just said. Using a doll, puppet, or stuffed animal can be another effective way to demonstrate what may occur.

Visualization and
Relaxation Exercises

Perhaps you can't always protect your youngster from pain, but you can alter his perceptions of the procedures. Explain that chemotherapy and radiation, no matter how unpleasant, are friends, not foes, working to keep him alive. Instilling in kids a sense of control over their cancer often helps them relax, and one way to do this is to have them close their eyes and *visualize* the battle raging within their bodies.

A favorite example reverses the premise of Chapter One's "Pac-Man" analogy for explaining cancer to children. Here the tiny video-game creatures represent chemotherapy or healthy white cells that rummage through the body, devouring the bad cancer cells. In another often-used imagination exercise your youngster pictures them as white knights come to vanquish the evil invaders. Or he imagines the drugs literally melting away his tumors. The possibilities are endless.

Does practicing these mind-over-matter techniques actually kill cancer cells? Directly, no. Studies into just how and why our psychological state affects our health are as yet inconclusive. But scientists believe certain strong emotions can trigger hormones that may curb pain, inflammation, and congestion as well as mobilize the disease-fighting white blood cells. Jason devised his own personalized mental image, which we'll tell you about in the next chapter, and it really helped him get through painful treatments.

Other visualization exercises for alleviating stress before or during procedures involve mentally transporting oneself to another place. Though there are several ways to achieve this relaxed state, here is one you can work on with your youngster:

1. Lie down or sit comfortably, limbs outstretched and joints loose, so as not to restrict circulation.

2. Close your eyes and take three deep breaths, releasing tension as you exhale.

3. Concentrate on thoroughly relaxing muscles from head to toe by squeezing each tightly and then letting go. Feel the peaceful, heavy sensation traveling down the body.

4. While continuing to breathe rhythmically, imagine a tranquil, comforting setting, such as a warm beach. Switch on all the senses: feel the soft breeze, hear the tumbling waves, smell the salty air, see the sailboats in the distance, and so on, until the scene seems real.

This becomes your child's safe haven, to which she may escape anytime. Naturally, depending on age and inhibitions, some youngsters incline more to this than others. Eventually your child may come to direct his own vivid scenes. Perhaps his idea of an oasis is lying in front of towers of amplifiers while his favorite hard-rock band shatters the sound barrier. To each his own, so long as it works.

Music can help stir the imagination. Many bookstores and libraries carry specially recorded tape cassettes of soothing music. Some may also feature a calming voice offering hypnotic suggestions. If you can't find these cassettes in your area, the Cancer Hot Line in Kansas City, Missouri, loans them free. Send a self-addressed, stamped envelope requesting a tape to Cancer Hot Line, 4410 Main Street, Kansas City, Missouri 64111, (816) 932-8453.

Hypnotherapy

Hypnotherapy is the treating of disease through *hypnosis,* a method of artificially inducing patients into a trance state during which they become susceptible to suggestion. Approved by the American Medical Association, hypnotherapy has been successfully used to control youngsters' pain awareness, anxiety, depression, insomnia, and nausea or vomiting.

For example to a child afraid of needles the hypnotherapist might suggest imagining her hand immersed in ice. She would then be instructed on how to recall that numb feeling during her next I.V. insertion. Or a child plagued by constant nausea could be guided into a trance and taught to calm his stomach, a sensation he would then summon on his own when next receiving chemotherapy.

Be forewarned that this field is rife with unqualified practitioners. To locate a trained and licensed hypnotherapist, ask your nurse, doctor, or social worker. Or contact the following organizations, either by sending a self-addressed stamped envelope for a list of professionals in your area or by calling for several referrals over the phone:

- American Society of Clinical Hypnosis, 2200 East Devon Avenue, Suite 291, Des Plaines, Illinois 60018, (708) 297-3317
- Society for Clinical and Experimental Hypnosis, 128A Kings Park Drive, Liverpool, New York 13090, (315) 652-7299

Biofeedback

Biofeedback utilizes a principle similar to hypnotherapy, training patients to regulate their reactions to treatment. However, in biofeedback the child is in a conscious state, wired to a machine that senses electrical current and indicates involuntary functions such as muscle tension with a flashing light or a beep. Through observing or listening to the machine, the youngster learns how to silence the signal by relaxing, until eventually the response becomes automatic. Biofeedback specialists are listed in the yellow pages under "Biofeedback Service." For free referrals in your zip-code area, call the Biofeedback Society of America, 10200 West 44 Avenue, Wheat Ridge, Colorado 80033, (303) 422-8436.

There may still be situations where no amount of preparation can spare your child discomfort, such as Jason's first bone-marrow aspiration. While Craig sat in front of him, not knowing what to expect himself, our little boy sprung forward from the excruciating pain, clawing at my husband's shirt.

Craig recalls, "He was looking at me as if to say, 'How can you let them do this to me?' What do you do? What do you tell him? You don't know what to tell him. After it was over, Jason was crying. I said, 'Go ahead and cry. I'll cry with you.'

"We did a lot of crying together."

Jason later said that aside from the bone-marrow aspiration and spinals, "the part I hated the most about having cancer was watching my mom and dad cry. Especially my dad, because I'd never seen him cry before. I guess it made me feel guilty, like, *Why am I doing this to these guys?*"

Craig and I shed buckets of tears during Jason's illness, believe me, but we tried our best to do so in private and to maintain as much optimism around him as we could. One night after chemotherapy my mother came into Jason's bedroom. I was sitting beside him, giving him water through an eyedropper. He was so sick and weak, half the time he brought it right back up.

Mom broke down crying. I don't blame her; it was a heartrending sight. Nevertheless I had to ask her to step outside. "Not here, Mother," I said. "Whether we're going to have Jason for a lifetime or six months or six weeks, I want that time to be as happy for him as possible."

My husband and I were determined not to turn our home into a tomb. There were going to be smiles and laughter, and should the worst happen, we were going to have happy memories to cherish. I'm not saying that parents have to act falsely cheerful. Kids will see right through you anyway. But sadness cannot incapacitate you. If we had lost control of our emotions, where would that have left Jason? Alone.

LOW-COST LODGING

For four of our five weeks in Rochester the kids, my mother, and I stayed in Northland House, located a few blocks west of the Mayo Clinic. A nominal-cost shelter, it was originally funded through physicians, church groups, and various organizations. Five years later Northland House joined the ranks of Ronald McDonald Houses, established by McDonald's Restaurants in 1974 as a home-away-from-home for patients and their families who must travel to obtain medical care. Since the first one opened near Philadelphia's St. Christopher's Hospital for Children, a hundred more have sprung up around the country and overseas, providing lodging for about 450,000 people a year.

As you can imagine, vacancies at the Ronald McDonald Houses, available on a first-come, first-served basis, are all too rare. We were able to spend nights there again only twice. To find out about the Ronald McDonald House nearest your child's treatment facility, ask the hospital social worker, who can help make the arrangements for you.

At the time of Jason's illness the sparsely furnished three-story Victorian house had just been restored and was cold and drafty. Years later we returned for a visit and could hardly believe our eyes. The outside had been painted a sunny, inviting yellow, and the inside transformed. It was beautiful, with modern kitchen facilities, plush carpeting, hanging plants, and plenty of entertainment for the kids, such as videocassette recorders.

Yet even in its former state, we were so thankful to be able to stay there. Besides the obvious convenience, Northland House made it possible for our family to maintain a semblance of normalcy and for Tim, Adam, and Melissa to be with their brother. Jason's doctors advised that a separation would traumatize them more than witnessing episodes of vomiting and so on. Had we been forced to check into a motel, it would have ruled out their coming to Rochester. No way could we have afforded putting everyone up for a full month.

Each family gets its own bedroom and shares a kitchen and dining room with the other three or four families on their floor. Guests are expected to do their own cleaning, grocery shopping, cooking, and laundering, these tasks coordinated and supervised by a full-time house manager. The nightly cost per family varies between five and fifteen dollars, depending on ability to pay. For those who cannot afford to donate, the lodging is free.

On days when Jason had only his radiation treatment, we were often back at Northland House by 9:30 A.M. Adam and Tim would play outside on the jungle gym; Jason, too, if he felt up to it. My mother, the baby, and I mostly sat around talking to other parents, which I found enormously comforting.

In Chapter Ten we write about the value of support groups. The other parents at Northland House *became* my support group. Pediatric cancer is such an isolating experience. I could talk to another mother in the neighborhood, and we'd have child-rearing in common, but the issues in her life would be completely different from those in mine. At Northland House everyone truly understood my feelings, because they were sharing the same experience, the same emotions. Plus, from the other mothers I picked up priceless advice on disciplining a sick child, which medicines caused sore throats, what to feed a kid with a poor appetite (malted milk shakes), and other tips.

We met some interesting people there, like a Jordanian diplomat whose teenage son suffered from osteosarcoma, and made wonderful friends. Another thing I found was that staying at Northland House helped to put our troubles in perspective. No matter how bad Jason's condition, we always encountered a youngster whose was worse.

Craig found that extremely uncomfortable. "I didn't like that place," he admits freely. "First of all, after not seeing my family for a week, when I came to Rochester, I wanted to be alone with them, not share the living room with other families. But also, everything would be going along well for us, with Jason making progress. Then I'd listen to another father tell me how everything had gone great for his kid, too, but a year or a year and a half later the child relapsed.

"I'd leave there feeling sick. Maybe I just didn't want to admit that Jason was like those other children, bald and sick-looking, but I don't see where staying there did me any good. I'd just as soon have been with my family in a motel." It goes to show that everyone is different, with different needs.

A FATHER'S BURDEN

Sometimes I think a child's cancer is almost harder emotionally on the father than on the mother. In most families the husband is still the primary breadwinner. As a result he may feel left out and and less informed, for it's often the wife who establishes the closer rapport with the medical team. I know I couldn't have gone to work every day the way my husband did, not knowing what was happening in Rochester, waiting for someone to call.

"It was tough," he reflects. "I thought about Jason all the time. *All* the time. It just keeps running through your mind. I'm sure I wasn't always the easiest person to get along with at work. If my wife said she'd try to call at a certain time and couldn't because there was a delay at the Mayo Clinic, I'd think, *Is something wrong? What are they finding out today? Is there another tumor somewhere?* I always worried that I'd get a phone call and Jason would be gone, that I'd never see him again.

"I was the new guy at work, and everybody would ask, 'How's your boy?' They were all concerned and tried to be as comforting as possible. But nothing really helped. To be honest, after a while you get tired of being asked, 'How's Jason?' Because you don't know. I'd come home from work to an empty house, have a bite to eat; it was nothing for me to lie down on the couch and doze off. Then I'd wake up hours later and crawl off to bed.

"I felt alone."

CHAPTER SEVEN

HOME FROM
THE HOSPITAL

Living with Pediatric Cancer • Disciplining Young Patients • Giving Medicine at Home • Discussing Death and Dying

The second week in August Jason's doctors pronounced him finished with radiation. So that Saturday we gratefully piled into the van and returned to Worthington. "It was great to get out of there after five weeks," remembers Jason. "You can't do anything, and it gets really boring." Stating the obvious, he adds, "I don't like hospitals."

When we pulled up in the driveway, Craig burst out the front door to greet us. He seemed somewhat shaken by Jason's appearance, which in the space of just a week had deteriorated drastically. I look at photos from that time, and the transformation is startling: his face grew gaunt and pale, the eyes and cheeks sunken, while the potbelly he developed taking prednisone weighted down his otherwise emaciated frame. The few remaining strands of hair on his head waved pathetically in the summer breeze.

"It was hard to look at him when he first got out of the van," Craig admits, "because he'd changed so much. He *looked ill*. To be honest, I had to walk away for a moment and collect myself."

The euphoria parents typically feel upon their youngster's discharge soon fades once they realize that being back home is by no means the same as being back to normal. I'd say I felt more relieved than joyful on that drive home from Rochester. A knot in my stomach told me that a so-called ordinary life did not await us.

One of pediatric cancer's less obvious effects is that it cancels your ability to plan for the future. I'm not talking about twenty years down the road, I mean not being able to organize an upcoming weekend because your youngster's blood counts might drop or he might run a fever, sending you rushing to the doctor. The disease takes precedence over everything, placing everyone's life in limbo. You stumble from one day to the next, which is not a very pleasant way to live.

And yet, you know something? You adjust, until this utterly abnormal existence *becomes* everyday life. It took our family about ninety days to reach that point. In retrospect I see that my coming to terms with Jason's cancer proceeded in stages very much like those accompanying a loved one's death. Shortly after the diagnosis came denial, anger, and grief. I went through a few days of hysterical screaming, crying, and pounding on walls, followed by crushing sadness and anxiety. Then, slowly, you struggle back to your feet and move forward, step-by-step.

While hardly the ideal way to live, under these circumstances it is certainly the sanest. Not only is mapping out the future futile, but the ominous possibilities are too painful to consider. Instead be flexible. Accept that chaos will reign for a time and that old routines will break down.

The first week or two back in Worthington was a very quiet stay-at-home, gather-our-strength kind of time. Jason felt so weak and tired from the cumulative effects of radiation and the ongoing chemotherapy, he spent most of his days stretched out on the living-room sofa. The other boys would sit beside him, playing together with their Superman and Batman figures. That was about all the strength Jason could muster.

LIVING WITH A
DEADLY DISEASE

"If I could say just one thing to kids with cancer," Jason declares, "it'd be that just because you have cancer, it doesn't mean you're going to die. So don't stop doing the things you really love to do."

Cancer disrupts a child's life terribly; all the more reason that young patients should be permitted to live as normally as possible. It took me awhile to realize that.

My immediate reaction upon Jason's return home was to overprotect him. Had it been solely up to me, I would have locked him in his room, instructed him, "Don't move!" and vigilantly watched over him twenty-four hours a day. Fortunately my husband provided a much-needed balance, encouraging our son to pursue his favorite activities.

"If Jake wants to ride his bike, let him ride his bike," he'd say with a shrug. I worried he'd have an accident and bruise or cut himself. Craig and I saw eye-to-eye on most issues concerning Jason's illness, but not on this.

Craig feels I sometimes overreact when it comes to the boys' health. Maybe I do, but never obsessively. As you might have gathered, sports play a large part in our family's life and always has. If Adam complains of an aching knee from football, I grow concerned. Especially since Jason's cancer, I'm much more inclined to follow up on a health complaint. "How is that knee today? Does it still hurt?" Whereas my husband would say, "Ah, just shake it off." I sometimes kid Craig, "So long as the limb was still attached to the body, you'd tell him to shake it off."

You can probably imagine my displeasure, then, when Jason announced he wanted to try out for the YMCA flag-football team. "Are you some kind of nut?" I exclaimed. Jason was so scrawny then, his little arms resembled chicken bones. I pictured him running with the ball and *Ka-Boom!* But Craig, who coached the team, argued in favor of it.

During a discussion one night Jason sat on the floor, listening. Finally he spoke up, "Mom, you don't want me to play football because you're afraid I might fall down, hit my head, start bleeding, and die or something, right?"

"Yes, Jason, I am. I'm afraid you'll hurt yourself."

"Well, what's the point of living," he asked innocently, "if you don't get to do the things you like to do?"

It was as if somebody had conked me over the head with a brick. I realized that I was trying to change his habits not for his sake but for mine, to reduce *my* anxiety. And so I handed over the matter to Craig. "You love Jason as much as I do," I said. "You regulate what he can and cannot do."

My husband's philosophy was to view our son's disease as chronic, not terminal. If he got up in the morning and felt fine, then for that day at least he was treated like a healthy child. Life had to go on. Craig sat Jason down and explained, "Your body isn't as strong as it was, so you have to listen to it. If you feel like you have extra energy and can play sports, go ahead. But don't push yourself, and don't try to do something just to prove that you can. If you feel tired, sit on the sidelines and watch." Which is exactly how Jason approached it from then on.

He remembers, "If Adam and Tim had friends over and I didn't feel good, sometimes they'd all come inside, and we'd do things that I could do: sort baseball cards, build models, play board games, color, do puzzles, watch TV. And then other times they'd play football outside. I used to watch them through the window and pretend to be the announcer, yelling, 'A touchdown for Tim!' and stuff like that.

"When I had cancer and played my sports, I wasn't too good. Like, in basketball, most of my shots didn't even reach the rim of the basket. Tim did most of the scoring; I barely got the ball because I couldn't dribble straight. So I went on to football. I guess they also thought I wasn't any good. I couldn't run or throw the ball, I was so weak, and whenever they passed to me, I dropped it."

Since Jason didn't have enough energy to run pass patterns, during team practices he stood next to his quarterback father and received the ball back from the other boys, handing it to Craig. The important thing was that he stayed involved. Jason's enthusiasm for sports had always exceeded his ability a bit anyway. Perhaps that's why he still enjoyed participating despite not being able to play up to par.

A kid used to excelling in a particular endeavor, be it athletics, academics, or whatever, may grow frustrated, his self-worth suffering in the process. It's up to parents to reassure a child with cancer that he is still the same person he was before he got sick, and that people are ultimately judged by who they are, not solely by their accomplishments.

Continuing to take part in sports gave Jason something pleasurable to look forward to, a welcome distraction from his disease and the rigors of therapy. In addition it helped him to build self-confidence and self-reliance, form friendships, and, most important, feel like a "normal" kid. Children uninterested in athletics should still be encouraged to keep fit to the extent that their stamina allows. Of 251 cancer patients responding to an Ohio State University study, 93 percent said they felt better physically and emotionally from exercise.

Your child's physician will discuss with you which activities are off-limits. One ironclad rule you can generally count on is no contact sports whenever the platelet count is low because of the risk of uncontrolled bleeding. Should you have to impose restrictions, tell your child why they are necessary and for how long. Then help him find alternate activities, such as inviting friends over to draw and paint, play board games, watch videos, or make crafts.

From the beginning Jason refused to accept the role of patient. He insisted he could do many of the things he used to, and by God, the little guy was usually right. One late-summer afternoon I prepared a comfortable spot for him on the living-room sofa, turned on the TV, and brought him a bowl of ice chips to suck on, for he was still lethargic and suffering painful mouth blisters from radiation. In short I got him all set to be safely bedridden for the day. Then I went about my housework.

When I returned to check up on him no more than a half hour later, Jason had disappeared, along with his ice chips. I frantically searched the house, then ran outside and down the block. From an adjacent lot I heard children playing ball, and there at shortstop crouched Jason, his thermos of ice chips in his back pocket. Between pitches he nonchalantly whipped out the thermos, took a nip of ice, and stuck it back in his pants. He'd been feeling better, he later explained, and saw no reason to loiter around the house all day. There was just no keeping him down, particularly once his strength returned.

Yet for a six-year-old Jason showed surprisingly good sense. You undoubtedly know what a chore it can be to get kids in bed, especially if there's a good TV program on. Some nights when we'd all planned to watch an eight o'clock movie, I'd come into the living room with bowls of popcorn and ask, "Where's Jason?" We'd look in his and Tim's room and find him sound asleep, the covers drawn up tight. Nobody had to tell him, "You're looking pretty droopy, it's time for bed." He instinctively knew his limits.

Those favorite activities he could still participate in, we did extra often. More than anything, Jason adores swimming and boating, so that summer we bought into a lakefront resort in Okoboji, Iowa, about forty-five minutes from Worthington. Financially speaking, Craig and I had no business whatsoever doing this. But knowing how much our son enjoyed the water, and not knowing how much time he might have left, we felt it was well worth the gamble.

I'm convinced that encouraging Jason to pursue the joys of childhood during these years was a factor in his emerging from cancer so well adjusted. And I have to wonder what effect my original inclination to treat him like a fragile flower—fixating on his weaknesses instead of his strengths—would have had on his spirit and self-image.

DISCIPLINING A CHILD WITH CANCER

Once home, children may behave in one of two extremes: regressing emotionally or acting aggressively. Thumb sucking, baby talk, or bedwetting are ways for a youngster to reclaim the attention received in the hospital, while a kid who flagrantly misbehaves may be seeking to reassert the independence surrendered there.

Young people with cancer have the same needs as before; not only love, care, and support, but discipline. Parents must insist on acceptable behavior and personal responsibility appropriate to their child's age. And they must impose limits, which all kids need to feel secure. That may be even more true of children with cancer. A patient whose parents suddenly overindulge him and no longer enforce household rules may think, *They're treating me differently; I must be dying.*

Admittedly it's easy to cave in to a sick child's every whim, to compensate for her misery. "That happens a lot," observes Ginny Rissmiller, the Mayo Clinic's pediatric-oncology social worker. "If your child is in the hospital for, say, a tonsillectomy, perhaps he gets spoiled for a few days, but then he comes home and things return to normal.

"With pediatric-cancer patients the overindulgence can persist for years. From the beginning we try educating parents about the importance of discipline, because hopefully the child is going to do well, go beyond treatment, and return to a normal childhood." Repeatedly catering to a youngster, she says, is likely to produce one spoiled, difficult cancer survivor.

At Northland House we came into contact with several couples who had obviously lost control of their children—one reason, in fact, that Craig objected to staying there. "Some of those kids got away with murder," he recalls. "I worried about the influence it might have on Jason." One pint-size terror was allowed to run roughshod over his entire family, issuing threats and throwing things if his incessant demands weren't met. What really struck me about him was that he seemed like such an unhappy little boy. Our goal in disciplining Jason was for him to be normal and happy.

From the outset Craig vowed to treat him no differently than the other boys, while naturally making exceptions for his unique situation and needs. Though Jason has always been well behaved, he, Tim, and Adam occasionally got into trouble and had to be punished. My husband once came home from work to find their room an unparalleled mess. In addition to the wrinkled clothes strewn all over the floor, the trio had stashed chewed Halloween candy and gum behind their dressers, leaving me a lovely wad of sticky gunk to clean up.

"What's going on here?" Craig demanded. "You boys have a servant to pick up after you? I think we need a little *attitude adjustment* in this house." That's Gaes lingo for a light spanking, something I realize not all parents believe in. Adam was the first to trudge downstairs to the basement, where he received three whacks on the behind. Next came Tim. Then it was his twin's turn.

By this time Jason weighed no more than forty pounds. Clad in just his underpants, he tottered down the steps on his spindly legs and assumed position.

"What do you have to say for yourself?"

"Well, Mom says I'm just like a pig, the worst of the bunch."

Whack, whack, whack. After Jason went back up to his room, whimpering, Craig stepped behind the furnace and cried his eyes out. "God," he said to me later, "that was the toughest thing I ever had to do." I nodded sympathetically. We both understood, though, that Jason was equally guilty and needed to be reprimanded along with his brothers. Had his blood counts been down that week, we would have devised another punishment, as kids with low blood counts should never be spanked.

"If we lose control of Jason now," Craig said, "we'll never get it back," and he was right.

In families of more than one youngster, spoiling the patient often creates another set of problems. As we discuss in Chapter Nine, healthy siblings endure their own considerable fears and anxieties during a child's cancer. Seeing their brother or sister lavished with affection and gifts may stir up resentment and jealousy. Naturally parents can't help but devote more attention to the ill child, and this should be explained early on to the other children.

I probably should have told Adam and Tim, "For a while your dad and I may not always get to spend as much time with you as we'd like. That doesn't mean we love you any less. But until Jason gets well, he needs our care more than usual, just as you would if you were sick." Parents can further mute rumblings of favoritism by encouraging the patient to share his booty and to respect his siblings' feelings. But don't be surprised if an overindulged child's cooperation proves less than spectacular.

We were lucky in that our sons were used to sharing with one another. Besides subdividing a bedroom, they liked trading clothes. If Jason's uncle Mike bought him a new toy, we never had to say to him, "This is for you and Tim and Adam." It was accepted that it belonged to all three. Jason would exclaim, "Boy, look at what we got. Wait'll I show Tim!" Always *we*, not *I*.

The only visible display of brotherly jealousy I ever observed was the time that Dan Marino of the football Miami Dolphins sent Jason a team warm-up jacket, just like the ones the players wear. The famous quarterback, an idol of all three boys, had read Jason's book and wanted to do something special for him. When the box arrived and Jason pulled out the striking aqua and orange jacket with the number thirteen emblazoned on its front, Adam's lip began to quiver.

"Nothin' that good ever happened to me in my whole life!" he whined.

"Adam, whadaya crying for?" Jason said impatiently. *"You're gonna wear it first.* Then Tim." His brothers practically wore the shine off that jacket before Jason finally slipped it on himself.

Tim now says, "I don't think I ever really felt jealous that Jason got all the gifts. I know I'd sure want presents if I had to get long needles stuck in my hand and back. I felt he deserved it, for doing what he had to and not quitting."

As with disciplining any child, mothers and fathers must consistently maintain a united front. Otherwise children will seek the path of least resistance, playing the more lenient parent against the stricter one. But what about well-meaning family members and friends? How do you prevent them from undermining your efforts not to pamper the patient? Grandmothers are particularly prone to spoiling ill youngsters. That's what grandmas are for. It's up to you to explain politely to others how you are handling disciplinary matters and to request that they abide by your wishes.

CARING FOR YOUNG PATIENTS AT HOME

I must confess to having conflicting feelings upon taking Jason home from the Mayo Clinic. Naturally I couldn't wait to reunite our family, but secretly I was terrified. At home there would be no round-the-clock medical care. I thought to myself, *I'm not a nurse. What if complications arise? Will we know what to do?*

Such apprehension is typical, according to Dr. Bringelsen, especially for families that live a distance from the medical center. "The hospital has become the parents' lifeline," she says. "We assure them that we would absolutely not send that child home unless we were certain that he was okay and that the parents could cope with whatever comes along."

Another common reaction is a changed perception of the patient. "Parents have expressed to me that the child they're taking home seems 'different,' " Dr. Bringelsen continues, "and that they don't know if they're capable of taking care of this 'different' child with all of his or her different needs."

Anticipating my nervousness, Jason's physicians offered words of encouragement. "You know your son better than anyone, Geralyn. You're plenty qualified to take care of him." They also reminded me that Dr. Faul, our Worthington pediatrician, had been copied on all of Jason's medical records. Before I left Rochester, they handed me a detailed two-page list of instructions outlining which medications my son could and could not take, symptoms to observe, and when to call.

The National Cancer Institute advises reporting any of the following conditions immediately:

• A fever of over 100 degrees Fahrenheit (taken orally), other signs of infection, or if the youngster just doesn't "look well"

- Exposure to a contagious infection, such as chicken pox or measles, even if you suspect your child might be immune due to previous exposure or vaccination
- Pain, discomfort, or chronic headaches
- Difficulty walking or bending
- Painful urination or bowel movements
- Reddened or swollen areas
- Severe nausea or vomiting
- Blurred or double vision
- Bleeding or multiple bruises
- Mouth sores
- Constipation lasting more than two days
- Severe diarrhea

Don't hesitate to pick up the phone for fear of "bothering" the physician. According to Dr. Smithson, "When parents leave the hospital for the first time, I tell them, 'We expect a lot of phone calls and questions, especially the first few months. Don't worry, just call.' " And so I did, at all hours. Social worker Ginny Rissmiller emphasizes, "We'd rather have parents call us anytime rather than worry until morning, since the child may need prompt attention, and care is critical."

The normal tendency among parents, she's found, is to overreact initially. "If we say, 'Watch for fever,' that doesn't mean to put a thermometer in a child's mouth every hour. You handle it the way you normally would, taking the child's temperature when he feels warm." Dr. Burgert says that most parents "gain confidence once they see their child is getting along pretty well and is back to his usual tricks."

Dispensing Medicine at Home

The first rule of giving any medicine at home is: *give it!* As directed. On schedule. Always. Remarkably the rate of noncompliance among teenage chemotherapy outpatients may be as high as 60 percent, and among younger children, between 18 and 30 percent, staggering figures that portend potentially tragic consequences. As Dr. Burgert gravely points out, "It's been shown that treatment has sometimes failed when patients did not take their tablets."

Considering what's at stake, to me this degree of negligence borders on child abuse. Yet few mothers or fathers who let their youngster occasionally skip medication would probably think of themselves as endangering that child. During *remission*, a temporary or permanent condition when no disease is detectable, the child's healthy appearance may lull parents into complacency and denial. *He doesn't look sick,* they reason. *I guess it wouldn't kill him to miss one dose.* Would you want to take that risk?

Or, wanting to spare their child the unpleasant side effects of chemotherapy, they let sympathy overwhelm common sense. Another frequent excuse is that the pill-taking schedules are confusing, which indeed they can be. For example, after each biweekly cyclophosphamide treatment Jason had to be given prednisone four times daily over the next several days, in tapered doses.

So that his schoolteacher wouldn't have to administer the pills, I volunteered as a classroom aid. Sometimes my son would be involved in an activity and ask if he couldn't wait until lunch. "No, Jason," I'd say, "we have to take it now." You can't be lax about this. Children must receive the precise dose at the proper time, no matter how inconvenient. To keep track of his irregular regimen, which included assorted antibiotics to combat infection, I kept a chart in my journal. Color-coding the various drugs on a calendar is another suggested method.

For younger children, pills can be crushed to a powder and mixed with a tablespoon of applesauce, jam, pudding, chocolate syrup, or other sweet foods. Nurse Betcher gave me a cuplike implement for administering Jason's prednisone. You filled it with liquid, set the tablet in its specially designed holder, then tipped it forward so that the liquid ran down the child's throat, carrying the pill with it. For some reason we could never get it to work properly. Jason would reopen his mouth, and the acrid-tasting prednisone would be stuck to his tongue. In exasperation he finally grabbed the pill from me, chewed it, and washed it down with juice. End of ordeal.

We had better success dispensing his liquid Benadryl and Phenergan, using another device from the Mayo Clinic. This one consisted of a small cylinder with a spoon-shaped top that rested on the child's tongue to prevent gagging. You doled out the medicine according to markings on either side of the cylinder (in both centiliters and teaspoons/tablespoons) and, again, let the liquid drizzle down the child's throat.

Medicines may also be delivered rectally, in the form of suppositories, or intravenously, either through a catheter or with a needle. Before releasing my father, diagnosed with prostate cancer, the Mayo Clinic nursing staff instructed me on how to inject his daily dose of leuprolide acetate.

Since kids generally associate taking medicine with feeling sick, they may want to know why they must take their pills when they feel fine. Explain that cancer cells may still be hiding in their bodies and that the chemotherapy is necessary to root them out and destroy them.

Can you entrust an adolescent to take medication on his own? Some want to, to feel like an adult—it is, after all, their body—and to take an active role in their recovery. Ultimately this is your call; you know your teenager's level of responsibility better than anyone. Should you decide to allow it, monitor him to ensure that he takes his drugs correctly.

RETURNING TO ROCHESTER

Every other week for over a year and a half, Jason and I made the nearly four-hour drive to Rochester for his outpatient chemotherapy treatments. Minnesota's weather is highly unpredictable, so during the winter months we left after school and spent the night at a motel on the outskirts of town. To eliminate the extra expense of lodging, in summer we took off around three in the morning.

Either way most of the trip was made in darkness along Interstate 90, a desolate stretch of road at that hour. One of the few landmarks, a radio tower bearing the blinking message JESUS IS LORD told me we were in Blue Earth, the midway point. As we cruised past southern Minnesota's farm country, there was little else to focus on except for the green metal markers counting off the miles.

The first several months' car rides were fairly tense. While my son slept, I wondered whether today we would receive some terrible news. Thus far Jason seemed to be progressing well. But as Craig observed earlier, you could never quite forget those harrowing stories of kids who appeared to be sailing smoothly toward recovery, only to be capsized by an unforeseen storm.

Sometimes Jason slept the entire way, not opening his eyes until I pulled onto the Mayo Clinic parking ramp. Other times he woke up just as the sun peeked over the horizon. Invariably the closer we got, the quieter and more nervous he became. Then came the nausea, usually right before the Rochester exit. I'd pull over, and Jason would get out and throw up.

Doctors have a tongue-in-cheek expression for this conditioned response: "parking-lot syndrome." I used to bring along an empty ice-cream carton for Jason to clutch whenever he felt sick, as well as paper towels, mouthwash, and screw-top bottles of 7Up to settle his stomach.

Toward the end of my son's therapy I learned that the American Cancer Society sometimes provides drivers or reimburses families for travel expenses to doctors' offices and treatment centers. We received some financial assistance, as has my father, who must travel to the Mayo Clinic for checkups. To learn what services your region's chapter may offer (baby-sitting, for instance), call (800) ACS-2345 or ask your hospital social worker. He or she can also inform you about other transportation options, typically available through the American Red Cross, and various religious and community organizations. The Leukemia Society of America's Patient-Aid Program (800-955-4LSA), too, reimburses qualifying families for up to $750 of transportation costs.

If treatment must take place far from home, you should be aware of Corporate Angel Network (CAN) and AirLifeLine, two nonprofit organizations that fly ambulatory patients and their parents to medical centers most anywhere in the country at no cost. Your hospital social worker can tell you if your child meets their criteria, which differ from each other slightly. For instance AirLifeLine requests proof of financial necessity, whereas CAN does not.

Several commercial airlines run similar programs, although the Mayo Clinic's Ginny Rissmiller cites CAN and AirLifeLine as "the two that really help." However, as you can imagine, coordinating the logistics of these air trips is complicated, and neither CAN nor AirLifeLine can guarantee an appropriate flight. For more information, contact:

- AirLifeLine, 116 Twenty-fourth Street, Sacramento, California 95816, (916) 446-0995
- Corporate Angel Network, Westchester County Airport, Building One, White Plains, New York 10604, (914) 328-1313

At seven o'clock my still-queasy son and I rode the elevator up to the Mayo Building's twelfth floor, where between fifty and sixty patients receive outpatient chemotherapy daily. Our agenda rarely varied from appointment to appointment, consisting of a blood test or complete blood count (CBC), ultrasound, body imaging, a physical exam, and then the drug treatments, with a good deal of waiting in between.

Considering the strain gripping many of the parents there, you'd have expected grumbling and occasional angry outbursts when waits stretched to several hours. To the contrary, I think most of us felt relieved. Having to wait meant your youngster's condition was stable enough not to be designated an emergency. If we had to sit for an hour and a half, it was because another child was sicker than Jason. With a shudder I'd think back to our first visit in June when *he* was taken ahead of all the others.

There wasn't much for kids to do in the quiet, carpeted waiting area, Jason remembers. "No TV or video games, just toys for real little kids, like teddy bears and stuff." To alleviate boredom, he suggests bringing from home some of the following:

- Toys
- Tape-cassette player, *with headphones*
- Pocket games, puzzles, playing cards
- Magazines, books, coloring books
- Stamp or photo albums
- Supplies for crafts, such as drawing, sewing, knitting, crocheting, macramé
- If your doctor permits, juices and healthy snacks

One other diversion, conspicuously absent from Jason's list: home-work.

Besides helping to pass the time "bringing fun things to do keeps your mind off throwing up." But nothing—probably not even a surprise visit by Dan Marino—could have prevented Jason from retching before spinals, especially if he had an hour or two to fret.

Every appointment we saw many of the same faces, the parents and patients forming a close-knit community. Frequently while the kids occupied themselves, we mothers congregated to quietly share recent developments. Whenever discussing your youngster's health, remember never to reveal anything you haven't already told your child. A parent later remarks about it to her spouse, their boy or girl overhears them, and before you know it the information, by now distorted, has filtered back to your child, with damaging results. Be discreet.

DISCUSSING DEATH AND DYING WITH YOUNG PEOPLE

A young patient's death casts a heavy pall over the pediatric-oncology floor. You'd step off the elevator and immediately sense something was wrong. Unfortunately about half the kids we met at the Mayo passed away. When you've known these children and have followed their progress and setbacks, each tragedy hits home hard.

In Chapter Two we introduced Jill, a lovely, pixieish little thing who also suffered from Burkitt's lymphoma. For the first year or so we ran into her and her mother regularly, and she and Jason became close friends. However, once Jill was declared in remission, their treatment schedules diverged, and we saw one another less and less. As soon as my son and I arrived on the floor, I always asked about Jill. My heart sank the day a nurse informed me that she'd *relapsed,* the cancer having reappeared. I knew that with each reversal the disease grows more indomitable and difficult to control. Yet the last I'd heard, Jill was getting along pretty well.

So I wasn't prepared for Dr. Burgert's response to my usual inquiry one morning. "Jason," he said distractedly, "would you please fetch me a pencil and pad from the nurse's station?" Jason merrily went on his errand, eager to be of assistance. Dr. Burgert gently closed the door to his office, cleared his throat, and in a subdued voice told me that Jill had died at home. Once it became apparent that chemotherapy could no longer stave off the lymphoma, he said, the doctors and her parents mutually agreed to discontinue treatment. Nurse Donna Betcher had gone home with the family to tend to Jill in her final days.

Only six years old, I thought, devastated. I had to hide my tears, though, because just then Jason appeared in the doorway.

For a day or two afterward I grappled with telling him that his friend had died. The more I thought about it, concealing the truth seemed dishonest. And, realistically, he was bound to find out eventually. So I made up my mind that once the side effects from the chemotherapy faded, I would sit him down and tell him.

Jason's reaction stunned me. "Where did she die?" he asked breathlessly.

"What do you mean, honey?"

"Where? Was she in the hospital, or did she die at home?"

"Well, she died at home."

"Oh, good," he replied, appearing almost relieved.

"Good?"

"Because," Jason explained, "the last time I saw her, she told me, 'I sure hope I can die at home and don't have to go to the hospital.' "

I thought back to that day, a few months before. While Jason had kept his friend company in one of the outpatient chemotherapy rooms, her mother and I stepped out into the hallway.

"Things just aren't working," she confided tearfully.

"Does Jill know?"

"Oh, my God, no! We don't know how to tell her or what to say."

But the little girl knew. Of course she knew.

Some well-meaning parents choose to ignore the prospect of death in the belief that they are protecting their sick child. It does seem almost cruel to broach such an awful subject with one so young and innocent. Yet many children with even a vague awareness of death are perceptive enough to sense that their illness is serious and possibly fatal.

"In the beginning," Jason remembers, "I thought about dying all the time."

He was full of questions that needed answering. During the first snowfall after his diagnosis, he couldn't sleep and gazed outside at the soft white carpet covering the ground. Wandering into the master bedroom, he asked, "Mom? When you die, and they bury you, do you get cold?"

I slipped on a robe and accompanied him to the living room, where we sat down to talk.

Naturally everyone's interpretation of death differs in accordance with their religious and spiritual beliefs. I explained it to him in a way I felt a young boy could understand.

"Well, Jason," I began, "to answer your question, I think that our bodies are very much like turtle shells. You know how a turtle crawls along, and then one day all that's left is the shell? That's how it is with us. When we die, what's good and unique about us goes on to another place, while the useless shell is left behind. So, no, you don't get cold, because the part of you that's *you* isn't there."

Jason nodded, appearing satisfied. For the moment at any rate. Throughout his illness he had countless questions, such as "What is dying like?"

I related it to when I was pregnant with him and his brother. Two weeks past my due date the obstetrician had to induce labor. "Before you and Tim were born," I said, "you didn't want to come out of my belly. I guess you liked it in there. Now that you're out, would you want to go back in my belly?"

Jason looked appalled. "No, of course not!"

"Why not?"

"Because it's so much better out here."

I said to him, "Well, I think heaven is very much like that."

Jason still remembers my words: "Mom said, 'Once we get to heaven, we won't want to come back here. We're just scared about going to heaven because we've never been there. In heaven you can see your grandpa again, and pretty soon your mom and dad will be there too. And then Tim and Adam, because's everybody's got to die some-time.' "

To dismiss a child's concerns—"Oh, you shouldn't worry about that, dear"—may only make death seem more frightening. By our being open with Jason, he came not to fear death, envisioning heaven as a place where the dearly departed engaged one another in basketball. He once remarked to my mother, "Grams, wouldn't it be fun if Uncle John and Jesus played me 'n' Grandpa Gaes in a game of hoops, and we beat 'em?" We all have our own concepts of the afterlife, but I dare say only the mind of a small boy could have hatched that one.

How to broach a topic as complex as death depends upon a young-ster's maturity. Between ages three and five, children first develop a vague awareness of death as something that happens to *things:* a pet, a bug, and so forth. They do not yet comprehend either the inevitability or the permanence of death, believing that they will live forever and that the deceased will one day return. During the early school years those notions about mortality evolve until by age eleven or so young-sters gain the intellectual capacity to fully appreciate death's magnitude. In teenagers and preteens fears of dying overshadow earlier anxieties about abandonment and bodily harm.

Parents must mind their language when discussing such a sensitive subject, for kids often take what we say literally. A young mind may interpret "Dying is like going to sleep" to mean that those who die *wake up*. Trying to comfort a child by saying, "Grandpa is watching over you from heaven," may inadvertently transmit the frightful image of a spy in the sky. A child told "We 'lost' your grandmother yesterday" may logically wonder when she'll be "found." And so on. To ensure that your message has been fully understood, it's always a good idea to have your child explain to you what she has just learned.

From an early age Jason has understood that death is a reality. Over the years he's asked to go to the funerals of several young friends who've died of cancer, and we've let him. While this might not be appropriate for all children, he found it to be a healing experience. Craig and I felt that it was important for our son to see that he, too, would be missed; that if anything happened to him, everyone who knew and loved him would gather and mourn his passing. Attending these youngsters' funerals also enabled Jason to be of comfort to others in their time of grieving.

When all efforts fail and a young cancer patient dies, the medical staff and the other parents often feel a double loss. That child's mother and father are no longer a part of the informal support network that binds parents of children with cancer. They vanish from your life just as abruptly as their youngster.

Sadly, after Jill's death, her mother and I drifted apart. I was now to her what the mother of a healthy child was to me: a woman who could sympathize but not truly understand. I'm not going to say I felt guilty that my son survived while her daughter died, but it was . . . uncomfortable for both of us. I didn't really know what to say to her. What I was thinking was *God, this is so unfair.*

"Everything looks great, Mrs. Gaes. We'll see you and Jason in two weeks."

The sky was usually darkening by then, ten or more hours after we'd arrived at the Mayo Clinic. With my son still woozy from sedation, I'd carry him out to the car, parked several blocks away. Following a spinal, patients must remain absolutely prone, and it was always tricky maneuvering my keys out of my coat pocket without raising Jason's head.

Once back in the car I'd exhale a deep breath of relief. *Whew, made it through another one.* In fourteen days the cycle would resume, touching off my fears again, but until then I'd take heart in the doctors' encouraging words. *Everything looks great.* At that moment, indeed, everything did.

Before getting back on the interstate, I'd stop off to buy my son containers of orange juice, to get fluids into his system, and a sandwich, Twinkies, and chips—whatever he felt like eating. Not the healthiest snacks, perhaps, but young patients deserve a treat at the end of a grueling day.

Several months of this—the fatiguing eight-hour round-trip drives, the apprehension, the pain of treatment, and the ensuing sickness— eventually wore down Jason's resolve. Once, on the way to Rochester, he asked me to pull over so that he could throw up. I got out and went around to the passenger side to help him. My little boy looked up and in a chillingly calm voice said, "Mom, I don't want to do this anymore. I'm tired of being sick."

"Jason," I said, trying to control my panic, "you know what will happen if we don't. We talked about this before."

"I know, Mom, but there's worse things than dying."

Aware that young children sometimes visualize death as a ghastly monster, I'd always tried to demystify the subject for Jason. Now I wondered if my approach hadn't backfired. "There's worse things than dying" is not what a mother wants to hear from her ill son.

Desperate, I asked him, "Jason, what can we do to keep you fighting? Something you want so much, it'll make all this worth it?"

He thought a moment.

"I want a party."

"A *party?*" Frankly I was expecting something more along the lines of "a pony."

"Yes," he replied. "I want a party where all the ladies wear new dresses and all the men drink beer."

I knew exactly what he was referring to. Earlier that summer Craig's youngest brother, Kirk, had married. It was an especially festive wedding. Several adults had whisked Jason out of his seat and danced him around the floor. He'd had the greatest time. And that's what he wanted, a reception in his honor.

"Honey," I said, smiling, "you've got it. As soon as your last treatment is over, the invitations go out."

From then until the end of therapy we used the party as a focus.

Whenever Jason felt scared, we put our heads together on his pillow, closed our eyes, and imagined the party: the guest list, the invitations, what everybody would wear, the food we'd serve. We planned the entire affair in our minds. I don't know how much it contributed to Jason's recovery, but fantasizing definitely made even the most uncomfortable treatments less stressful.

"It helped me during the spinals," Jason claims. "I'd curl up real tight, close my eyes, and think about the party I was going to get when I finished with all this."

CHAPTER EIGHT

DIET AND NUTRITION

Controlling Side Effects with Diet • Healthy
Snacks • Encouraging Kids to Eat • Vitamins and Nutrients

All parents try to ensure that their kids eat a balanced, nutritious diet. But when your child has cancer, that concern can assume overwhelming proportions. "If anything, we minimize the influence of diet," says Dr. Gilchrist, "because families can become obsessed. It's the one thing they have a certain amount of control over, or *think* they should have control over."

Compared with the many other ways you will be caring for your youngster, feeding her is the simplest, the most basic, and the most emotionally charged, for in our culture nourishing and nurturing go hand in hand. Add to this the current interest in the alleged health-ensuring qualities of food, especially when it comes to cancer, and it's easy to see why many parents become needlessly anxious about their child's nutrition.

You can achieve a well-rounded diet without emptying out your refrigerator and pantry or converting to a rigid health-food diet. The key is to understand how nutrition works and what's in the food your child enjoys eating, and then strive for a balance.

Because children's bodies are still growing, good nutrition is essential, better enabling them to withstand treatment and to recover from cancer. The irreparable long-term effects of poor nutrition on their development during this time can result in weight loss, weakness, a compromised immune system, and lack of energy.

Throughout your youngster's treatment it may seem that everything conspires against good eating: from therapy's disagreeable side effects to your own inability to put three square meals on the table every day. The cancer itself can stunt the body's absorption of food nutrients while at the same time hiking its caloric demand. Then, of course, all parents are familiar with their kids' sometimes bizarre eating habits.

Each child is different, and your physician may issue strict guidelines about your youngster's diet. During certain treatments and over time her nutritional needs may change. Feel free to discuss with your doctors or the hospital dietitian any concerns you might have. And needless to say, if your child has been prescribed a specific diet—for example, preceding surgery—follow it to the letter. Later in this chapter we'll examine special diets and ways of helping to ameliorate therapy side effects with food.

THE BASICS OF NUTRITION

Our bodies' life-sustaining processes are supported by substances called *nutrients:* proteins, carbohydrates, fats, vitamins, minerals, and water. Few foods contain adequate amounts of all six, and many processed foods contain none at all. That is why understanding what's in the food your child eats is as important as seeing to it that he does eat.

We are truly a calorie-conscious society, but calories and nutrients are not the same thing. Calories are the body's fuel. Once converted into energy, they make possible normal body functions such as growth and development and all forms of physical activity.

A child with cancer requires extra calories to maintain his stamina. While it's not necessary to count every calorie, you should be aware of approximately how many calories your youngster consumes. The labels on most packaged foods contain this information, while any bookstore or library has several titles listing the caloric and nutritional content of foods.

The following chart of recommended daily calories for children from infancy to age eighteen is reprinted from an informative booklet titled "Diet and Nutrition: A Resource for Parents of Children with Cancer," available free from the National Cancer Institute (800-4-CANCER). Bear in mind that these amounts are for *healthy* youngsters, who do not require as many calories as those suffering from cancer.

	Weight (pounds)	Height (inches)	Calories Required Daily
Infants			
0–6 months	14	24	702
6 months–1 year	20	28	972
Children			
1–3 years	28	34	1,300
4–6 years	44	44	1,800
7–10 years	66	54	2,400
Boys			
11–14 years	97	63	2,800
15–18 years	134	69	3,000
Girls			
11–14 years	97	62	2,400
15–18 years	119	65	2,100

As you can see, a child between ages seven and ten has roughly the same caloric demands as a teenage girl. And most children over seven burn more calories than a grown woman. To increase calories (and protein) in almost any food you serve:

• Add butter to hot foods such as mashed potatoes, soups, cereals, vegetables, and rice
• Top off desserts and warm drinks with a dollop of whipped cream
• Dried fruits can add substantial calories to hot or cold cereals

• Make dips for vegetables and chips with fat-rich sour cream, cream cheese, or protein-dense beans
• Sprinkle chopped or slivered nuts on vegetables, cereals, and salads

When a child's appetite waxes and wanes, snacks assume special importance. Fortunately many of the foods kids like to munch on, such as cheese, ice cream, nuts, seeds, fruit, and fruit juices, are nutritious. Even pizza has its place in healthy eating. Other nourishing snacks include:

• Cream cheese
• Gelatin salads
• Muffins
• Creamed soups
• Hard-boiled or deviled eggs
• Raw vegetables
• Cakes and cookies prepared with whole grains, fruits, nuts, wheat germ, granola
• Sandwiches
• Desserts

• Crackers
• Buttered popcorn
• Milk
• Cottage cheese
• Peanut butter
• Cheese cake
• Cereals
• Yogurt
• Milk shakes
• Applesauce

Meeting your child's protein and calorie needs is a top priority, and if she finds nothing appetizing but vanilla ice cream and chocolate syrup, so be it. Calories are calories, and provided a young patient isn't suffering other nutritional deficiencies, there's no harm done.

WHAT NUTRIENTS DO AND WHERE TO FIND THEM

Protein

The body uses protein and its constituent amino acids to build and maintain body tissues; to form enzymes, antibodies, and certain hormones; to regulate body processes; and to supply energy. Of the six nutrients, only protein can build and repair body tissues. Many people erroneously consider protein-rich foods prime sources of energy. In fact *carbohydrates and fats* are superior energy sources. Your child must receive enough of these so as not to waste valuable protein on energy production.

Best sources:

- Meat (especially pork, beef, veal, lamb)
- Poultry (especially chicken breast)
- Dried beans and soybean products
- Frozen yogurt
- Pumpkin, squash, and watermelon seeds
- Peanut butter
- Eggs
- Cheese
- Fish (especially seafood)
- Peas
- Lentils
- Milk
- Ice cream

Carbohydrates

Carbohydrates, starches, and sugars replenish energy. What the body doesn't need right away is stored, while the balance is converted to fat, which the body can break down for energy later.

Best sources:

- Bread, cereals, flour products
- Rice
- Sugar, honey, syrups, jelly
- Corn
- Popcorn
- Nuts, seeds
- Noodles and pasta
- Grains
- Potatoes
- Peas and beans
- Fruit
- Pretzels
- Pizza

Fats

These supply essential fatty acids that carry fat-soluble vitamins needed for bodily functions. Fats are also a concentrated energy source, supplying, ounce for ounce, twice the calories of protein or carbohydrates. A teaspoon of butter, for example, has double the calories of a teaspoon of jelly (carbohydrate) or yogurt (protein). While this makes fat the bane of most people's diets, it is a godsend for young cancer patients.

Best sources:

- Butter, margarine, oils
- Mayonnaise
- Peanut butter
- Meat fat (as in gravies)
- Fatty meats (especially sausage, ham, marbled meats, luncheon meats, hotdogs)
- Cream cheese
- Ice cream
- Cheese
- Nuts
- Whole milk
- Cream
- Olives
- Sour cream
- Chocolate
- Avocado

Vitamins

Vitamins—organic substances derived from plants and animals—serve many important functions, among them helping the body to process other nutrients and to form blood cells, hormones, and nervous-system chemicals. Yet humans need only a small quantity of vitamins. If distilled and measured, the average daily requirement would amount to less than an eighth of a teaspoon.

Excessive quantities of some vitamins can be dangerous, even toxic, for young cancer patients. Unless your doctor specifically prescribes a supplement, do not give your child any vitamins, not even the over-the-counter daily variety. A healthy diet can provide virtually all the vitamins your child needs.

There are two types of vitamins. *Fat-soluble* vitamins (A, D, E, and K) are stored in body fat and therefore are not required every day. *Water-soluble* vitamins (eight B vitamins and vitamin C), on the other hand, must be replenished daily.

Fat-Soluble Vitamins

Vitamin A is necessary for normal vision, to keep the skin and inner linings of the body healthy and resistant to infection, and for bone and tooth development. The foods we eat provide vitamin A in two different forms. One, *retinol,* is found in animal foods, such as whole milk, butter, egg yolk, cheese, and liver. The other, *beta carotene,* comes from dark-green, deep-yellow, and deep-orange fruits and vegetables.

Best sources:

- Whole milk
- Egg yolk
- Yellow vegetables (summer squash)
- Green, leafy vegetables (especially spinach, kale, collards, and turnip and beet greens)
- Liver
- Pumpkin
- Vegetable-juice cocktail
- Butter
- Whole-milk cheese
- Broccoli
- Apricots
- Cantaloupe
- Peaches
- Carrots
- Sweet potatoes
- Tomatoes
- Mangoes
- Papayas

Vitamin D is necessary for strong bones and teeth. While exposure to sunlight naturally produces vitamin D, parents must ensure that children who are largely confined indoors get enough.

Best sources:

- Milk and other milk products fortified with vitamin D
- Best of all: the never-popular cod liver oil
- Tuna
- Margarine
- Egg yolk
- Salmon

Vitamin E aids in the formation of red blood cells, muscles and tissues, and prevents the destruction of other nutrients, including vitamin A.

Best sources:

- Vegetable oils (coconut, corn, olive, palm, peanut, safflower, sesame seed, soybean)
- Whole-grain breads and cereals
- Green, leafy vegetables
- Wheat germ
- Nuts
- Liver
- Corn
- Dried beans

Vitamin K enables the blood to clot normally.

Best sources:

- Green, leafy vegetables (spinach, kale)
- Peas
- Cereals
- Cauliflower
- Cabbage
- Liver

Water-Soluble Vitamins

Thiamine, vitamin B_1, enables the body to release the energy in food and to synthesize chemicals crucial to the nervous system. Growth, appetite, digestion, and healthy nerves, heart, and blood vessels depend on thiamine.

Best sources:

- Organ meats (liver)
- Whole-grain and enriched bread, pasta, and cereals (especially oatmeal)
- Nuts (especially pine nuts, Brazil nuts, pecans, peanuts, walnuts)
- Pork (especially ham, bacon, sausage)
- Beef
- Wheat germ
- Eggs
- Peas
- Lima beans

All living cells need *niacin, vitamin B_3,* to produce energy and form DNA. Niacin is widely found in plant and animal foods, and children's deficiencies are rare.

Best sources:

- Chicken, beef, and calf liver
- Fish (especially tuna, cod, swordfish, salmon, rockfish, mackerel, sardines)
- Whole-grain and enriched bread, pasta, and cereals
- Turkey
- Lamb
- Peanuts
- Milk
- Dried peas, beans

Riboflavin, vitamin B₂, assists in the growth and repair of tissues, DNA synthesis, and metabolism of other nutrients for energy. It is particularly important for healthy eyes, skin, and mucous membranes.

Best sources:

- Dairy products (especially milk, cheese, yogurt)
- Nuts (especially almonds)
- Duck
- Whole-grain or enriched bread, pasta, and cereals
- Dried peas, beans
- Liver
- Brewer's yeast
- Wheat germ
- Goose
- Eggs
- Pork

Pyridoxine, vitamin B₆, is needed for many things: growth, a healthy nervous system, regulation of blood glucose levels, and the formation of red blood cells. Some experts contend that Americans don't get enough vitamin B₆, so be sure to serve some of the foods below each day.

Best sources:

- Organ meats (especially liver and chicken liver)
- Nuts (especially filberts, walnuts, peanuts)
- Pork (especially ham)
- Currants
- Turkey and chicken white meat
- Potatoes
- Fish (especially salmon, tuna, mackerel, lobster, swordfish)
- Green, leafy vegetables
- (especially spinach)
- Peanut butter
- Sunflower seeds
- Prunes
- Dried apricots
- Raisins
- Bananas
- Soybeans
- Green beans
- Avocado
- Whole-grain cereals and bread

Cyanocobalamin, vitamin B₁₂, helps form red blood cells, maintain the nervous system, support growth, and synthesize DNA. Deficiencies in children are rare.

Best sources:

- Organ meats (especially kidneys and liver)
- Milk (especially nonfat dry milk)
- Seafood (especially shellfish)
- Liverwurst
- Liver pâté
- Meat
- Most cheeses
- Eggs

Folacin, folic acid, is vital for cell growth and red-blood-cell development.

Best sources:

- Green, leafy vegetables (spinach, turnip greens, collards)
- Asparagus
- Cereals
- Filberts, cashews, almonds
- Avocado
- Corn
- Sunflower seeds
- Soybeans
- Liver
- Brussels sprouts
- Beets
- Parsnips
- Dried beans, peas
- Wheat germ

Pantothenic acid aids in the synthesis of adrenal hormones and nerve-regulating substances as well as metabolism. Pantothenic acid is present in all plant and animal foods.

Best sources:

- Nuts (especially peanuts)
- Salmon
- Meat
- Most vegetables (especially dark-green vegetables)
- Liver
- Kidneys
- Eggs
- Milk
- Whole-grain cereals and bread

Biotin helps the body metabolize protein, carbohydrates, and fats.

Best sources:

- Peanuts
- Milk
- Most vegetables (especially dark-green vegetables and green beans)

- Liver
- Kidneys
- Egg yolk
- Meat

Ascorbic acid, vitamin C, maintains body cells (including those in bones and teeth), blood vessels, and connective tissues. It aids in healing wounds and resisting infection.

Best sources:

- Citrus fruits (oranges, grapefruits, lemons, limes, tangerines)
- Melons (especially cantaloupe)
- Green and red peppers
- Dark-green vegetables
- Cauliflower
- Cabbage
- Peas
- Cherries

- Strawberries
- Tomatoes
- Broccoli
- Potatoes
- Kiwi fruit
- Papaya
- Brussels sprouts
- Apple juice
- Blackberries

Minerals

Minerals are essential to good health. Fortunately the body requires such minute amounts that a balanced, nutritious diet usually meets all needs. Iodine, manganese, copper, magnesium, zinc, cobalt, and fluorine are called trace minerals because they are needed in even smaller amounts.

Calcium, found in nearly all body tissues, is critical to the formation of bones and teeth, blood clotting, regulating muscle contraction (including the heart's), transmitting nerve impulses, and several other key bodily functions.

Best sources:

- Milk
- Yogurt
- Collards
- Canned fish (mackerel, salmon and sardines) *with* bones
- Almonds, filberts
- Cheese
- Broccoli
- Kale
- Tofu

Phosphorus combines with calcium to form bones and teeth and is found in every cell, where it assists with metabolism and acid-base regulation.

Best sources:

- Milk and milk products
- Fish
- Poultry
- Meat
- Egg yolk
- Dried beans, peas

Sodium is found in virtually all body cells. Along with chloride and potassium it is an *electrolyte,* a mineral that maintains the body's crucial fluid balance. Most Americans eat more than enough sodium, largely because almost every food except fruit contains some of this mineral. Nearly all packaged and processed foods (canned soups, luncheon meats, cold breakfast cereals, condiments, and even desserts) contain "hidden" salt. For example we need only 220 milligrams of salt a day, a requirement easily met or exceeded by three Oreo cookies, two slices of Wonder Bread, or one ounce of American cheese. Sodium intake becomes a serious concern when your child experiences dehydration from severe vomiting or diarrhea, or simply isn't eating enough.

Best sources:

- Table salt added to food in cooking
- Bread
- Celery
- Pastry
- Cheese
- Salted nuts
- Hominy
- Sauerkraut
- Milk
- Pickles
- Carrots
- Olives
- Spinach

Potassium combines with sodium to help balance body fluids and is essential to the transmission of nerve impulses. Bouts of diarrhea and vomiting can quickly deplete potassium levels, and a severe imbalance can adversely affect the heart. For this reason *should a condition possibly leading to dehydration persist for more than a day or two, notify your child's doctor immediately.*

Best sources:

- Dried fruits (especially apricots, peaches, raisins, prunes, figs)
- Nonfat dry milk
- Pumpkin and squash seeds
- Potatoes
- Pork
- Swordfish
- Avocado
- Milk
- Bananas
- Wheat germ
- Oranges
- Almonds
- Peanuts
- Dry lima beans
- Turkey
- Sardines

Iron is essential for the formation of red blood cells, among other tissues. Yet it is estimated that perhaps over 80 percent of children between ages three and five do not receive the recommended daily allowance of this crucial mineral, readily available in a balanced diet.

Best sources:

- Liver
- Pumpkin, sunflower, and squash seeds
- Green, leafy vegetables
- Dried fruits (especially prunes, raisins, apricots)
- Enriched or whole-grain bread and cereals
- Potatoes with skin
- Red meat
- Egg yolk
- Wheat germ
- Sardines
- Codfish
- Dried peas, beans
- Turkey
- Chicken
- Molasses

Iodine is needed to form thyroid hormones, which regulate metabolism.

Best sources:

- Iodized table salt
- Seafood

We rarely think of *water* as a nutrient, but in fact the body needs water more than food. Water aides with digestion, excretion, temperature regulation, and countless other functions. It exists to a certain degree in almost all foods, particularly soups, juices, milk, fruits, and vegetables. A child's water requirement depends on her age and size. For example, a six-month-old baby needs about one quart of water a day and will likely derive most of that from her formula or milk. A six-year-old, however, may need double that amount. Your youngster's water intake becomes a serious concern when he is suffering from fever, diarrhea, or vomiting.

Fiber, which contributes roughage or bulk to the diet, is not usually considered a nutrient, yet it is no less important. Available in whole-grain breads and cereals, raw and dried fruits, nuts, and raw vegetables, fiber helps promote regular bowel movements. Your doctor may recommend additional dietary fiber if constipation is a problem. Conversely a child who suffers diarrhea or other intestinal problems might be placed on a low-fiber diet.

HOW CANCER AND CANCER TREATMENT AFFECT NUTRITION

A healthy child's body readily stores nutrients, conserves energy, and regulates metabolism. During brief illnesses it can compensate for a temporary reduction in food intake by redistributing nutrients to the most essential organs and functions.

Pediatric cancer, its treatment, and the resulting stress and exhaustion often impair the body's ability to store and use nutrients. Your child may not feel like eating, and what he does eat may not be absorbed or metabolized as efficiently. To reiterate a point made earlier, children are particularly vulnerable to nutritional deficits, because their bodies are still growing.

Anorexia, or appetite loss, is perhaps the most common side effect of cancer and cancer treatment. While the causes are not entirely understood, it seems likely that a variety of psychological, biochemical, and emotional factors, as well as drug and treatment side effects, play a role. Mouth sores, nausea, vomiting, altered taste, and other problems make food even less appealing.

Cachexia, severe weight loss and the wasting of body tissues, can occur from appetite loss or effects of the disease or treatment. If your child does not eat sufficiently, the body will compensate by breaking down muscle tissue, a process that is difficult to halt or reverse. You can avoid cachexia by ensuring that your youngster's diet provides sufficient calories and protein.

MANAGING SIDE EFFECTS THROUGH DIET

As seen in Chapter Five, the side effects of cancer and cancer treatment are many and far-ranging. But each child is unique. Yours may experience one of these side effects, all of them, or none. Similarly what succeeds for one young patient doesn't necessarily work for another. You'll probably discover the best solutions for your child through trial and error. Remember to listen to your child and above all be patient, for your anxiety over his eating habits may only make him more upset and resistant.

If your child has great difficulty eating and is losing weight, your doctor may prescribe a commercially prepared diet or dietary supplement. Most often these are specially formulated, fortified milk-shake-type products. Jason really liked them, especially chilled or blended with ice.

Nausea

Controlling nausea is vital to adequate nutrition and to help prevent vomiting. Here are some measures to take:

• Instead of serving three large meals a day, encourage your child to eat many small meals or snacks throughout the day.
• A stuffy, overheated room, or one that reeks of cooking odors or other

aromas, can contribute to nausea. If necessary, allow your child to eat his meals in another part of the house.

- At mealtime avoid serving liquids, which can make a youngster feel too bloated to eat. Instead, urge her to sip liquids throughout the day. Sometimes drinking through a straw also helps quell nausea.
- Serve beverages cool or chilled. Freeze favorite drinks as ice cubes, or mix juice and ice in the blender to make a slushy.
- Never force your child to eat if he feels nauseous, which may cause a long-term aversion to that particular food.
- Make mealtimes pleasant and leisurely.
- Activity can slow or hamper digestion, so set aside time after meals for your child to rest.
- Young people with cancer often feel at their best in the morning. If that's the case with your child, take advantage and serve high-protein, high-calorie breakfast foods, such as eggs, ham, buttered toast, milk, and cheese.
- Conversely if your child feels nauseous first thing in the morning, have her munch on dry toast or crackers before getting out of bed.
- Observe, if you can, a pattern to your child's nausea. Are there certain foods, surroundings, or events that seem to induce queasiness? Once you can pinpoint a possible cause, rearrange your child's diet or eating schedule.
- Foods that tend to soothe nausea include vegetables; fruits; baked or broiled skinned chicken; sherbet; pretzels; angel-food cake; dry food, such as toast and crackers; salty, low-fat foods, such as pretzels; and cold foods.
- Those that often exacerbate nausea include fat; greasy or fried foods; overly sweet foods; spicy, hot foods; and anything with a strong aroma, such as certain types of fish.
- Alert your doctor to any changes in your child's eating habits, especially severe, recurrent nausea.

Vomiting

If your child vomits:

- Withhold all food and liquid until the vomiting has subsided.
- Following a vomiting episode reintroduce food gradually. Begin with

a teaspoon of clear liquid every ten minutes: broth, clear soup, consommé, tea with lemon and sugar, flat carbonated beverages, tomato juice, strained vegetable broth, fruit-flavored juices, strained fruit juices, lemonade, limeade, fruit ices without milk or fruit chunks, or plain gelatin. Then work up to a tablespoon every twenty minutes, and finally to two tablespoons per half hour.

- While on clear liquids, avoid bread, cereal, flour, cheese, desserts (except plain gelatin), eggs, fat, meat, poultry, fish, legumes, milk products, potatoes, rice, and pasta.
- A clear liquid diet will not meet nutritional needs, only maintain bodily fluids. If your child has difficulty digesting clear liquids, contact your physician.
- Once your child can tolerate the clear liquids, gradually begin serving *full* liquids, also in small increments. Full liquids include those clear liquids mentioned above as well as refined or strained cooked cereals for gruels, soft or baked custard, sherbet, plain cornstarch pudding, plain yogurt, ice milk, smooth ice cream, butter, cream, oils, margarine, all fruit juices and nectars, small amounts of strained meat in broth or gelatin, skim and whole milk, milk shakes, chocolate milk, buttermilk, potatoes pureed in soup, cream soups, and strained or blended soups.

Diarrhea

Diarrhea has a number of causes, including chemical or bacterial toxins, infections, drugs, abdominal radiation, food sensitivity, malabsorption of nutrients, and emotional and psychological factors. Certain cancer therapies can produce lactose intolerance, which results in the body's incomplete digestion of milk and milk products and diarrhea.

Severe or prolonged diarrhea is a potentially serious problem that should be brought to your doctor's attention at once. It depletes body nutrients by rapidly eliminating fluid and minerals. Nutrient absorption is impeded by the food speeding through the digestive system. Suggestions for managing this condition include the following:

- Try the "small amounts frequently" method previously outlined for both liquid and solid foods.
- Twelve to fourteen hours after a bout of acute diarrhea, serve clear

liquid foods. This will replace essential body fluids without taxing or aggravating the bowel.

- Gradually move from clear liquids to full liquids and then to soft foods low in fiber, roughage, and bulk:

Refined white and seedless bread
Biscuits, rolls
Refined cooked or ready-to-eat
   cereals
Ice milk, ice cream, sherbet, ices
Any type of egg but fried
Vegetable shortenings and oils
Commercial French dressing
Bananas
Canned or cooked apples
Grapefruit and orange sections
   without membranes
Tender beef, lamb, veal or liver
   that is baked, broiled,
   creamed, roasted or stewed
Seedless grapes
Roasted or stewed pork, chicken,
   duck, turkey, cornish game
   hen
Cooked, fresh, or frozen fish
   without bones
Crackers
Pancakes, waffles
Mild cheeses
Custards, gelatins
Butter, margarine

Cream
Mayonnaise
Sour cream
Juices, nectars
Avocado
Apricots
Cherries
Peaches
Pears
Tuna fish
Almonds
Creamy peanut butter
Dumplings, noodles
Brown or white rice
Spaghetti
Potatoes that are baked, boiled,
   creamed, scalloped, mashed,
   or au gratin
Mashed sweet potatoes
Canned or cooked asparagus,
   beans, carrots, beets,
   eggplants, mushrooms,
   parsley, pumpkin, spinach,
   squash
Tomatoes, tomato juice,
   vegetable-juice cocktail

- Milk and milk products can produce diarrhea in children with lactose intolerance. If you suspect this is the case, discuss it with your physician, who may recommend low-lactose milk products, available in most supermarkets, or enzyme tablets and drops that aid in the digestion of dairy products.
- Try foods low in fiber, such as fish, chicken, tender or ground beef, eggs, pureed vegetables, canned or cooked fruit without the skin, ripe

bananas, cooked cereal, smooth peanut butter, and bread made with refined flour.

• Avoid greasy, fatty, or fried food; citrus juices; carbonated beverages; raw vegetables and fruits; cooked vegetables that are high in fiber (broccoli, celery, cauliflower, corn).

Constipation

Constipation has a number of causes: anticancer drugs, lack of adequate dietary fiber or bulk, insufficient exercise, obstruction or intestinal spasm from emotional stress or irritants. Here are ways to prevent and cope with constipation:

• Encourage your child to drink lots of liquids. Have a wide variety on hand.
• Having your youngster drink a hot beverage around the time he normally moves his bowels can stimulate a bowel movement.
• Bran is an excellent source of fiber. Add it to homemade bread, casseroles, cookies, and breakfast cereal.
• High-fiber foods include whole-grain bread, cereal, and pasta; brown rice; fresh, unpeeled fruits and vegetables; popcorn; dried beans; oatmeal cookies; and corn chips.

Sore Mouth, Gums, or Throat

Not surprisingly, a child plagued by any of these side effects will be even more reluctant to eat. When radiation had left the inside of Jason's mouth painfully blistered, he favored cold items, such as milk shakes, frozen fudge bars, and bland soft or liquid foods, like his grandpa's potato soup. Experiment with these suggestions to make chewing and swallowing more comfortable:

• Serve soft foods such as mashed potatoes; custards; scrambled eggs; ice cream; bananas; peach, pear, and apricot nectars; watermelon; cottage cheese.
• Puree foods in a blender.
• Encourage your child to drink through a straw.
• Food may be easier to swallow if cooked until soft and tender; cut into small pieces; or served with butter, thin gravies, and sauces.

- Piping-hot foods may burn or irritate tender tissues. Serve meals more at room temperature.
- Among the foods to avoid are tomatoes; citrus fruit and fruit juices (orange, grapefruit, tangerine, lemon, lime); spicy or salty foods; rough, coarse, or dry foods, such as raw fruits and vegetables, granola, toast, popcorn, corn chips, and tortillas.

Altered Taste, Loss of Taste

This side effect, also known as *mouth blindness,* can give food a strange, bitter, or metallic flavor, or no taste at all. It may take some experimentation to learn what will work for your child. For instance, while Jason was sick, he grew to love spicy tacos.

- Serve foods that look and smell appetizing.
- Drinking liquids with meals helps to counteract the disagreeable taste.
- Red meat, such as beef, especially tends to taste unpleasant. Chicken, turkey, eggs, dairy products, and fish are all equally good sources of protein.
- Unless your child has tender gums and mouth, offer tart foods such as oranges, lemon custard, and lemonade.
- Cold or room-temperature foods often taste better than hot.
- You can make chicken, meat, and fish more flavorful and appealing with marinades of sweet fruit juices, Italian dressing, or sweet-and-sour sauce.
- Enhance the flavor of vegetables with onions or minced bacon or ham.
- Season foods with strong herbs, such as basil, oregano, and rosemary, or lemon juice.

Dry Mouth

Dry mouth can also alter the taste of food as well as make it difficult to chew and swallow. Observe the tips below, which can also help with mouth and throat sores.

- Very sweet or tart foods, such as lemonade, limeade, or grapefruit juice, may increase saliva production and make swallowing easier. But

do not give your child acidic citrus foods if she has a sore throat or tender mouth.
• Puree foods.
• To make foods easier to swallow, top them with butter, gravy, sauce, or salad dressing.

Changes in Appetite

The chemotherapy drug prednisone frequently stimulates a hearty appetite. Once Jason's mouth sores healed, he began devouring everything in sight. And as Craig observes wryly, "He hasn't stopped since." Our son used to wolf down three substantial meals a day, all the while snacking in between. Then in the middle of the night he'd awaken me in bed complaining of hunger.

"Well, honey," I'd mumble, "there are some apples and oranges in the refrigerator."

"No, Mom, I'm *really* hungry. I want pork chops, corn, potatoes, and gravy!"

I'd get up and prepare it all for him or reheat leftover portions from dinner. Gladly, too, for our son weighed a mere thirty-five pounds then. Though we all grew used to his ravenous appetite, strangers were occasionally stunned to see this skinny little boy put away enough food to satisfy the entire Minnesota Vikings defensive line.

At a restaurant one time Jason ordered a four-piece chicken dinner that included potatoes, gravy, corn, rolls, and a big tumbler of milk. After he'd cleaned his plate, the waitress asked, "Is there anything else I can get you?"

Jason replied, "I would like to have one more."

"One more piece of chicken?"

"No, one more dinner!"

GENERAL SUGGESTIONS
FOR MAKING MEALS
MORE APPETIZING

When your child is ill, it's wise to relax family routines where meals are concerned. Some days she may eat breakfast, lunch, and dinner at the usual times; other days she may snack intermittently and not join the rest of the family. Whatever time she does decide to eat, encourage her to do so slowly. Coax, but never force, a youngster to eat.

Once you discover a pattern to your child's appetite, schedule his meals accordingly. When he feels like eating, don't stop him, especially if he faces upcoming treatment or surgery. Building up nutrient reserves now will help carry your child through those times when he cannot eat.

The appearance, texture, and presentation of food can influence a child's appetite. Garnishes of cheese cubes, crackers spread with soft cheese, deviled eggs, olives, or croutons add calories to foods in addition to enhancing their appeal. Also try introducing familiar foods in unique forms: string cheese and cheese sticks, different kinds of rolls and muffins, fun-shaped pastas, fruit rollups and "miniature" foods, such as Ritz Bits crackers.

Kids thrive on novelty. Remember how much better a breakfast cereal in the small snack packs tasted than the same thing out of the larger box? The next time you go shopping, why not let your youngster accompany you and pick out foods especially for him? You may return home with items you normally wouldn't purchase—animal crackers, dinosaur-shaped macaroni, pistachio instant pudding, Teenage Mutant Ninja Turtle breakfast cereal—but your child will undoubtedly look forward to mealtime more.

We tried to allow Jason as many choices about his life as possible. For a long time his favorite meal consisted of a hamburger and a chocolate malt, so that is what he ate two or three times a week. Not the ideal diet for a healthy child, true, but the combination well suited our son's nutritional needs, containing ample levels of protein, fat, and calories. He also took to orange juice, swigging it down with every meal. Only later did I discover that when consumed with iron-rich foods, the juice's vitamin C boosts the body's capacity to harness and absorb the iron.

While this is not the time to radically overhaul your family's diet or introduce too many new foods, experiment a little. A child who likes orange juice may also enjoy the taste of orange-pineapple or orange-pineapple-banana juice blends; raisin bran instead of regular bran cereal; or ground turkey or veal in place of conventional hamburger.

RECOMMENDED RESOURCE

• American Institute for Cancer Research Nutrition Hotline, (800) 843-8114, Monday through Friday, nine A.M. to five P.M. EST

A registered dietitian will answer any questions you have concerning diet, nutrition, and cancer.

CHAPTER NINE

CANCER'S OTHER VICTIMS

Effects on Siblings • Fathers • Mothers • Marriage
• Family Finances

If I have one regret about the way Craig and I handled our family's crisis, it was our failure to appreciate the impact one youngster's life-threatening illness has on the rest of the family. We were so preoccupied with Jason's condition then that I believed, *Tim is not sick, Adam is not sick. So long as their basic needs are met, they can coast along until we get Jason fixed up. Then we'll turn our full attention back to them.*

I've since learned that you can't put kids' emotions on hold. As my husband later told Tim and Adam, "Jason feels the pain of the needles, but we feel the pain in our hearts." I wish Craig and I had seen the truth of that statement from the very start.

Adam, Tim, and Melissa each reacted to Jason's cancer in ways as unique and different as their personalities. Missy, less than a year old when her brother was diagnosed, has no memory of him being sick. Yet she was every bit as affected as her siblings.

For her first ten months I was a nursing, stay-at-home mother, as I'd been for all three sons. Then Jason's cancer abruptly uprooted Mommy and consumed her attention, leaving much of Missy's caretaking to Craig and her grandparents. Although she appeared to adjust happily,

I was concerned that my daughter's infancy was not as secure and nurturing as those of our other children.

When she reached kindergarten age, Missy began throwing up every morning before school. Yes, separation anxiety is normal in youngsters departing the nest for the first time, but I couldn't help wondering if it was related to her unsettled earlier years. Although the vomiting subsided, Missy is more clinging and babyish than the boys were at her age. This could also be because she's the youngest child (a girl with three doting big brothers). But I can never totally discount the feeling that my absences during her babyhood were a factor.

Despite the reigning tumult of those years Melissa was a joy—a laughing, playful baby who provided refuge from uneasy thoughts of death. "If anybody helped me get through that time," says Craig, "it was Missy." On days when there was little to smile about, she cheered everyone up, including Jason. If he were lying on the sofa, pale and nauseous, Missy would crawl over and plant a drooly kiss on her brother's nose, eliciting a laugh as he wiped the trickling "goober" off his face.

I now know that I really missed the boat with Adam, who on the surface seemed to accept quietly the turmoil at home. As the oldest and most independent of the boys, he shouldered far more responsibility than you'd imagine your average eight-year-old could. Craig leaves for work at five-thirty in the morning, so if Jason and I were gone to Rochester, it fell to Adam to make his younger brother and sister breakfast, shepherd them through their morning rituals, and escort Tim to the school bus. He did all this without a word of complaint, and I doubt a mother could have been prouder.

It wasn't until after Jason's recovery that Adam let on he'd sometimes felt neglected and resented the attention bestowed upon his brother. He also reluctantly admitted, "At night I used to get into bed, pull the covers up over my head, and cry myself to sleep." When we heard this, Craig and I were astounded. Not only hadn't he expressed those feelings to us then, but his behavior never hinted that anything was troubling him. In addition to helping run the household, he maintained good grades in school.

"At first I felt a little resentful," Adam admits. "But then I realized there was no way I'd change anything. I saw what Jason had to go through, and I sure wouldn't have wanted to trade places with him. So I felt bad about feeling jealous.

"One of the hardest things about Jason's cancer was to know that my mom and dad were hurting. That was *real* hard. There wasn't much I could do, but I wanted to help out as best as I could, making meals and doing the laundry and stuff."

Had I known it upset Adam when I couldn't attend one of his football games because his brother wasn't feeling well, I could have gotten my mother to look after Jason and slipped out of the house for a few hours. I just assumed Adam understood why I couldn't be there the way I had in the past. In hindsight—why is everything so much clearer in hindsight?—I would have observed Adam more closely, to better assess his needs. Today he advises kids whose brother or sister has cancer, "Let other people know what you're feeling, that it's hurting you, too, not just the person with cancer."

Tim also bottled up his feelings. But with Jason's twin it was glaringly apparent from the start that he was suffering and would need extra love and attention. He and Jason have always shared an almost symbiotic kinship that is unique even for twins. Especially before they entered adolescence, their identities were virtually interwoven. So one of them having a chronic disease was bound to devastate the other.

Tim reacted with horror the first time he saw his brother bald. "Jason came walking downstairs with no hair and a towel wrapped around his head," he recalls. "I thought it was a stranger! Not only was it scary watching him throw up and everything, it made me real sad. I wondered why it was him." It doesn't take a degree in psychology to understand that for Tim seeing his twin visibly ill was like viewing his own reflection, and this clearly terrified him.

Earlier I wrote how the boys were so inseparable that as babies they sucked on each other's toes while sleeping in the same crib. Once we moved them into their own cribs, I'd tiptoe into their room and find them clutching each other's fingers through the slats. Even as little boys the two of them used to snuggle up against each other in bed like a couple of spoons.

But with the onset of Jason's lymphoma, Tim suddenly began avoiding his brother. He simply could not believe that he didn't have cancer himself if his brother did. *Jason and I have always done everything together and are so much alike,* he reasoned. *What if I have these things growing inside of me, only nobody knows it?*

"When Jason got cancer," he recalls, "I refused to get in the same bed as him anymore. My mom would find me on the floor or on the living-room couch. I'd make up different excuses: 'I fell out of bed.' Or 'I must have walked here in my sleep.' And I wouldn't wear the same clothes as Jason like we'd used to, because I was afraid I'd catch his cancer. It kind of made me feel guilty."

At the same time Tim acted anxious whenever his brother was out of sight. One of my most painful memories is of the day Craig and I had to take Jason to the Mayo Clinic for therapy. My mother and father were staying at our house to take care of Adam, Tim, and Missy.

As the car started down the street, Craig glanced in the rearview mirror and saw Tim running after us, frantically screaming, "Don't take him! Don't take him!" He and Jason had never involuntarily been apart before, and Tim was convinced he'd never see his brother alive again. Craig promptly turned around and drove back to the house. "Get 'im ready, Grandma," he told my mother. "We're taking Tim with us."

LETTING SIBLINGS
WITNESS TREATMENT

At one point Dr. Burgert suggested that both Tim and Adam might benefit from observing Jason's treatment, to better understand what their brother went through. After all, what could two young boys possibly imagine after hearing us discuss such alien terms as *chemotherapy* and *spinal?* It hadn't occurred to me that either might be interested in actually seeing it. But when I asked them if they'd like to accompany Jason and me next time, Tim and Adam chorused, "Sure!"

So the two of them stood gaping from the doorway as Jason's doctor prepared his spinal injection, then plunged the syringe into his back.

"I'm kind of glad I saw it," Tim now says, "but when I *did* see it, I kind of wished I wasn't alive. Just watching Jason get that big needle stuck in him made a quiver go up my back. I started to cry. And hearing him scream, that was really bad. Adam and I had to plug our fingers in our ears."

The scene so upset Tim, he ran crying down the hall. I trotted after him, calling his name, and finally found my son whimpering inside a broom closet. While Adam reacted as I'd hoped, coming away with a newfound respect for his little brother, Tim was traumatized by what he'd seen and withdrew even more from Jason.

Obviously, letting Tim witness his sibling's treatment did not achieve the desired effect. Nevertheless I believe this approach is worthwhile for many youngsters. When weighing its benefits and drawbacks, parents must take into account their child's age and emotional makeup. Perhaps if we'd walked Tim through Jason's chemotherapy, radiation, and so forth back in the early stages, before he'd constructed such elaborate fantasies about the procedures, it would have calmed rather than exacerbated those fears.

That summer Tim began stuttering. Interestingly the impediment seemed more pronounced whenever his brother was around, to the point where you could barely understand him. At the suggestion of the boys' schoolteacher, we took Tim to a therapist. The condition, she felt, was plainly related to the stress at home and symptomatic of a little boy who couldn't—or wouldn't—express his emotions.

My son's reluctance to divulge his feelings left me perplexed. Why was he holding back?

I soon discovered the reason. Both Tim and Jason were enrolled in a private Catholic school that held a children's mass every Friday. I liked to attend myself. As I walked down the aisle one morning, I glanced across the church at Tim, surrounded by his classmates. All the kids were on their feet, voices raised in a hymn, but Tim just stood there, tears rolling down his cheeks. I took his hand, gently led him out of the church, and drove him back home.

"Timmy," I said, "you have got to talk about this."

"I can't."

"What do you mean you can't?"

"Because," he said, "every time I talk about Jason, *you start crying!*"

I was dumbfounded. Tim apparently felt that he had to bear his burden alone because Mom had enough on her mind. *He* was trying to protect *me*.

I explained that it was okay to cry, that it was an expression of a feeling and made us feel better, and told him in no uncertain terms that he held no responsibility for my tears. After that, and with the help of the therapist, Tim began to open up, confiding how afraid he was of "catching" Jason's disease and how fearful he became every time we took his twin to Rochester.

SIBLINGS' OTHER COMMON REACTIONS, ANXIETIES, BEHAVIOR

Understandably brothers and sisters of a child with cancer can feel neglected, abandoned, or insecure about their place in the family. Their silent cries for attention may manifest in the following ways:

- Complaints of psychosomatic illnesses, such as headaches, stomachaches, or fatigue
- Babyish behavior
- Bed-wetting
- Undereating or overeating
- Undersleeping or oversleeping
- "Perfect" behavior
- Poor performance in school
- Refusal to attend school
- Aggressive, defiant, argumentative behavior

It's not unusual for kids who are cooperative and supportive at home to release their frustrations in school. I'd advise conferring with your healthy child's teacher from time to time, to learn of any disruptive conduct. We had the opposite problem with Tim. A model student in the classroom, at home he was prone to crying jags and temper tantrums. I mentioned this to his therapist, who said she considered it a positive sign that our son felt free to express himself around us yet apparently understood that such behavior was unacceptable elsewhere.

Other reactions to be mindful of:

- Guilt. Taunts of "I wish you were dead!" sometimes return to haunt siblings of a child with cancer. Tim once remarked with remorse that he'd shoved Jason at a carnival, as if that had caused his brother's cancer. Guilt-ridden youngsters must be reassured that nothing they did, said, or thought brought about their sibling's condition.

- Embarrassment. Youngsters, so eager to fit in among their peers, may avoid bringing friends home out of embarrassment over their ill sibling's appearance, believing it reflects negatively on them.
- Fear of their parents' sorrow. "It was tough to see my dad cry," recalls Tim, "because I'd seen him cry only once before, when Grandpa Gaes died. It made me feel real . . . *odd*, like *This is really bad; Dad doesn't cry very much.*" I went to my bedroom and started crying myself because I couldn't stand to see my dad, the big macho man, in tears."
- Fear of the patient's dying.
- Anger at the parents, for "allowing" their brother or sister to get sick.
- Feeling uninformed about their sibling's condition.

While there is no simple way to allay a sibling's stresses, many of the suggestions in Chapter Six on comforting young patients apply here as well. Basically, healthy youngsters require a great deal of parental support and love. They also need to feel included in what is a full-family crisis.

As Adam made clear a few pages ago, siblings, too, can suffer from the helplessness that pediatric cancer imposes on all members. Encouraging kids to cheer up a sick brother or sister, or to share in household chores—whatever they can readily handle—enables them to regain a semblance of control. At the same time, you're enhancing their self-esteem and instilling a sense of belonging, so crucial when many youngsters feel isolated and alone.

I don't believe you can shield a sibling from the reality any more than you can the patient herself. Children are quite sensitive to their family's concerns and will eventually piece together parents' unbridled tears and snippets of overheard conversations to form a fairly complete—if somewhat distorted—picture of what is going on. Craig and I recommend that when discussing the patient's condition with your other children, withhold as little information as their ages, maturity, and understanding of disease warrant, but be careful not to alarm them unnecessarily.

At six Tim knew enough about cancer to ask periodically, "Jason could die, couldn't he, Mom?" He was obviously hoping to hear in reply, "No, he's not going to die, Tim." For many months I could not say that without offering what would be false reassurance. If the worst actually happened, what then? Instead I'd say, "Yes, but he's doing well, and his doctors are very encouraged." Tim needed to hear the truth, no matter how difficult it was to face sometimes.

Whenever you can, spend time alone with each child. Listen to his concerns and fears. Take a special interest in his activities and accomplishments. Reiterate why you can't be as involved in his world right now as you'd like and that it's all right for him to feel resentful on occasion. We say this with the realization that any parent presently coping with children's cancer is probably thinking, *But my time and energy are stretched to the limit already.*

This is where grandparents can be a priceless asset (a subject explored in greater depth in the next chapter), by compensating for your diminished time. When Craig and I were away with Jason, my parents often stayed with the boys. "Grandma and Grandpa Lanham showed us a lot of attention," recalls Adam. "They'd come over, help us around the house, do the laundry, and take us out to dinner. They really helped me and Tim through it."

Compared with when Jason was ill, today's health-care system is far more attuned to the emotional and psychological fallout a child's cancer rains down upon his brothers and sisters. Some medical facilities have formed peer-counseling groups expressly for siblings, where *their* feelings are the priority and they can talk freely about whatever's bothering them. Even a well-adjusted child may find comfort at these sessions. Your social worker can tell you about any in-hospital support groups, when they meet, and so forth.

The Candlelighters Childhood Cancer Foundation, an international network of parent groups, also sponsors auxiliary groups for teenage siblings. To get in touch with the Candlelighters group nearest you, call the organization's headquarters toll-free at (800) 366-2223 (202-659-5136 in Washington, D.C.) or ask your social worker. (See Chapter Ten for more information on the value of support groups.)

Suggested Reading for the Patient's Siblings

From the National Cancer Institute (800-4-CANCER):

• "When Someone in Your Family Has Cancer"

From the American Cancer Society (regional offices, 800-ACS-2345; national office, 404-320-3333):

• "When Your Brother or Sister Has Cancer"

PEDIATRIC CANCER'S EFFECT ON PARENTS

Thus far we've examined the impact a young person's cancer has on every family member but you and your spouse.

Let me elaborate on an opinion expressed earlier. Pediatric cancer often exacts a greater emotional toll on husbands than on wives. Perhaps it's somewhat different in other areas of the country, but with men still the main wage earners in most families, women usually assume the brunt of the young patient's care.

Dr. Smithson loosely estimates that 80 percent of the time he deals primarily with the patient's mother. "We have a saying," he says jokingly, "Women are strong, men are good-looking."

With this immense responsibility falling chiefly on the wife, how is it that the husband frequently suffers more?

For generations men have been discouraged from declaring their emotions, a cultural bias that has only recently begun to change. Again, I concede this may be more common in the rural Midwest, a stronghold of traditional values and male-female roles. But generally speaking, boys are still raised to cultivate classic masculine attributes such as strength and stoicism over tenderness and expressiveness, both considered feminine. The strong, silent type has long been an American male archetype. As a result, men may be unprepared for the emotional jolt of a child's catastrophic illness, acting confused, even ashamed, of the awkward new feelings that engulf them.

As husband, father, and breadwinner, Craig had always been the head of our household, the family protector. In ten years of marriage it seemed there had never been a single problem that he couldn't solve somehow. Now here was a crisis utterly beyond his control, and it was a bitter, painful pill for him to swallow.

Craig's masculine role model, his father, was a big-hearted but emotionally controlled man. "I think the first time my dad hugged me was when I was twenty-seven or so," he recalls. At family funerals Fred Gaes was the one who reined in his grief, comforting everyone. My husband assumed that in a similar situation, he would react similarly.

"But when it happened," he says, "I wasn't like that at all. I just went downhill. When we first learned that Jason had cancer, I figured it was my place to call the family and let them know. And the moment Geralyn's mother came on the line, I just froze. Later, standing in the hallway, I kept thinking, *You've got to get control of yourself. Dad would have barreled right on through this.*"

As I frequently reminded my husband, who's to say how his father would have reacted? He'd never faced the prospect of losing one of his sons. Nevertheless that incident deeply troubled Craig. Having failed to meet his high expectations of himself, he believed he'd let me down. *I* certainly didn't think that, and it was painful to watch him be so hard on himself, piling guilt upon grief, sadness, and anger. All because he hadn't measured up to some unrealistic male stereotype. How unfair.

My husband still wrestles with those feelings. "Geralyn handled Jason's cancer better than I did," he says. "She was the one who took the trips and wiped his vomit out of the car. She was so strong, and strong in front of me. The same as I tried to be strong in front of her. But I felt I'd let her down. Before, I thought I could withstand just about anything; I discovered that maybe I was weaker than I thought."

Craig has always been the quiet type. But following our son's diagnosis he buried his emotions to an extent that was unusual even for him. "He just didn't want to discuss it," my mother recalls. "If you asked, 'How are you, Craig?' or put your arms around him, he'd say, 'I don't want to talk about it.' And he wouldn't."

The abrupt change in my husband's personality was so readily apparent that concerned family and friends used to ask, "Is Craig okay?" Anybody who knew him well could see the strain.

"He felt lost," observes his mother, Lea Gaes, "like he didn't know which way to turn."

The less intimate nature of most male friendships may further handicap a father from coming to grips with his feelings. On the whole, women are more likely to ask a young patient's mother how she's coping than their husbands are to ask the child's father. Buddies will ask the dad, "How's your boy?" but not "How are *you*?" as male conversations tend to center on mutual interests rather than on innermost feelings. With his father gone, and not wanting to overburden his still-grieving mother, Craig felt emotionally abandoned, as do many fathers.

"Geralyn was my shoulder to lean on because I didn't have anyone else to talk to," Craig says. "She was my tree to sit under. She was everything."

My husband now understands that he was as great a source of comfort and strength for me as I was for him. I'm as verbal as he is reserved, yet I could always come to Craig with my joys, my reservations, my fears, and it was okay. He listened patiently and never belittled my concerns, even when I probably was "borrowing trouble," as we say, worrying needlessly.

I never doubted that the two of us could withstand this challenge. But then, no matter how strong you think your marriage is, how do you know if you've never been so rigorously tested before? I have to admit that at first I was somewhat tentative, wondering how much I could lean on this relationship. I soon realized that I could lean, jump, *swing* on this relationship. It was as solid as an oak. Craig and I emerged from Jason's cancer even closer, more open, and more sensitive to each other's needs.

Unfortunately that is not the case for all married couples. While lodging at Northland House, I met the family of a young boy just diagnosed with cancer. Two months later I bumped into the mother, this time alone with her son. "Where's your husband?" I asked.

"We're getting a divorce," she replied matter-of-factly.

"Oh, my God, at a time like this?"

"Well," she said, "this made me realize that our marriage had a lot of problems, and always did. My husband and I were constantly working at it for as long as I can remember. When my son got sick, I had to decide whether I was going to turn my emotional energy to salvaging our marriage or to caring for our little boy. I knew I didn't have the strength to do both."

Rarely do husbands and wives react the same way to a child's illness. This can prove advantageous, with one partner's strengths compensating for the other's weaknesses, and vice versa. Or it can magnify heretofore overlooked differences to such a degree that the marriage crumbles.

Take, for example, a not-uncommon situation that Craig and I found ourselves in: where the parent less involved in the day-to-day caretaking persists in almost fatuous optimism, at times evoking the other parent's resentment.

From the very first day at the Mayo Clinic, Craig held fast to Dr. Bringelsen's assertion that Jason was going to make it. "When she said that," he recalls, "something inside me clicked, and I never let go of it."

In retrospect that was probably a good thing; his optimism an anti-dote to my occasional spells of despondency. Sometimes, though, I felt that Craig was stubbornly denying the harsh reality. So when he would try to calm me by saying, "I just have this feeling Jake's going to be all right," occasionally I'd think, *But you're not submerged in what's really going on here! You don't see the whole picture: the side effects from treatment, the painful medical procedures, the other sick-looking kids.* I can see how this could cause friction in families where the responsibility for the patient was com-pletely one-sided.

Craig and I compromised, deciding that unless Jason's physicians told us otherwise, we would try our best to stay optimistic. *Cautiously* optimistic. Throughout this book we've emphasized the importance of maintaining hope, for the patient's sake as well as yours. However, it's a fine line between a sanguine attitude and outright denial.

Conflicts between couples may also arise when a partner—typically the one less involved in the child's care—withdraws, frequently escap-ing through work. This, too, is a form of denial. The father of a dying twenty-one-year-old patient we befriended at Northland House never came to visit her in the hospital, always claiming he couldn't get away from his job. The young woman underwent *five* lung surgeries, and each time the father found another excuse to stay away.

"It's not that he doesn't love us," her mother explained sadly, "it's just that he can't face the fact that his only daughter is going to die." One can only wonder about the guilt that man must have felt over emotionally abandoning his child, who after a valiant struggle passed away.

Despite Craig's and my contrasting dispositions, we achieved a healthy balance that benefited everyone, but most of all Jason. As we wrote about in Chapter Seven, given my druthers I'd have ball-and-chained our son to the house, whereas Craig insisted, rightly so, that he have a relatively normal childhood. I worried more and needed to express my feelings more than my husband did. Had we both been intense, verbal personalities, who knows what fireworks might have resulted?

I remember one time when I accidentally dropped a dish in the kitchen. It wasn't an heirloom or anything, just something I'd picked up in a dime store. I guess my nerves were as shattered as that plate, because I started bawling like a baby. Craig came in, put his arms around me, and said gently, "Don't worry about it. I'll clean it up."

MARRIAGE MAINTENANCE

A chronically ill child definitely monopolizes your time and attention, but couples mustn't neglect each other. Besides the obvious disadvantages, marital strife prevents parents from responding to the young patient's needs. It takes a concerted effort to keep a marriage thriving during this taxing time. Here are some suggestions:

• *If work schedules and the proximity of the medical facility allow, share in your child's health care.*   Parents can become virtual strangers when only one gets actively involved in their youngster's recovery. Ideally both partners should have relationships with the medical team and become familiar with treatment. When a child is hospitalized, try alternating nightly and weekend visits, so that the parent working full-time can feel included and his spouse can recharge or spend time with the other children at home.

• *Discuss matters other than your child's cancer.*   A youngster's life-threatening illness weighs so heavily on your mind, it sometimes seems like there's nothing else in the world to talk about. But parents spend so much time comforting others, they may lose sight of their own feelings. Take the time to talk privately with each other about what *you're* going through. Through sharing feelings, partners can reclaim common ground at a time when they may feel themselves drifting apart.

• *Don't avoid intimacy.*   As can happen at any point during marriage, two people's sexual desire for each other may not always be in harmony. A tragedy like children's cancer can stir the need for increased closeness. Or it can preoccupy one's mind, precluding sexual feelings. It's not unusual for one or both parents to avoid sex simply due to exhaustion or out of guilt, as if their deriving pleasure is somehow inappropriate. Speaking for myself, this was a time when I particularly needed to reaffirm the love in my life—to feel alive.

• ***Give yourselves a break.***   On those rare occasions when you can get away, do it, just the two of you. Go out to dinner, see a movie, check into a hotel somewhere. Take your mind off your sick child temporarily and concentrate on each other.

• ***Know what you're angry about.***   Those times when you vent frustration at each other, remember the true source of your anger: the disease.

• ***Find things to laugh about.***   Believe it or not, a child's pediatric cancer does have its occasional lighter moments. Even Jason, who seems to have inherited his dad's dry wit, could find something to laugh about. The week after he began cranial radiation, he was washing his hair. Out it came, in fist-size clumps. Our six-year-old calmly stepped out of the shower, wrapped a towel around his head, and wandered into the kitchen, where I was fixing lunch.

Straight-faced, he whipped off the towel and said, "Mom? I think you'd better buy a different brand of shampoo. This one's too harsh."

To preserve your sanity, you *need* laughter.

There's no way a husband and wife can come through a crisis like this unchanged. I know that in some respects I certainly am different from the woman I was prior to Jason's cancer, more independent and self-reliant.

When Craig and I married, we mutually agreed that I would stay home and raise the children. It was what I wanted to do. But I now see that my being a housewife and mother kept me insulated and overly dependent on my husband. Aside from driving locally, I'd never gone anywhere on my own. I couldn't read a road map or follow directions. Many seemingly insignificant things that most people take for granted were simply beyond me then. I laugh about it today. In a sense my somewhat sheltered childhood extended into adulthood, as I went directly from my father's home to my husband's. Ironically my mother had been a liberated woman long before women's lib, traveling on the road to train salesmen for the same company that employed my dad.

Jason's illness forced me to broaden my horizons and to rediscover Geralyn Gaes. I couldn't have imagined driving across Minnesota in the dead of night or asserting myself to the medical staff. Because Craig came from a very traditional home, initially my newfound self-confidence threatened him.

I don't feel like I've grown away from my husband, just grown up. That I no longer depend on him for every little thing doesn't diminish his importance in my life at all. Unlike some men in the same situation, Craig was secure and wise enough not to try repressing me or insisting things return to the way they were. He accepted that we'd entered a new stage in our relationship, one with different dynamics.

Craig also changed from this experience. On a practical level he, too, became more self-sufficient. He had to, if he wanted to eat something other than take-out pizza, tacos, and hamburgers. He learned how to cook, clean, do the laundry, wash the dog, shampoo Melissa's hair—whatever domestic tasks needed doing while I was away.

He says about me, "I discovered that Geralyn is a very strong person." And I learned that just because Craig is a man of few words doesn't mean he is a man of few emotions. In the past I'd sometimes misinterpreted that reserve as timidity. But I came to realize that he is very strong, very sure of himself, and a solid decision maker. I look at him with renewed admiration and appreciation.

I now see Craig bringing up his sons very, very differently from the way his father had raised him. One time Adam felt embarrassed because he'd cried about something. I heard my husband say to him, "Hey, we're real people in this house, not macho men. I've got feelings, you've got feelings, and you've got a right to cry if you want." *Gee,* I thought, *is that my Craig?*

THE FINANCIAL COST
OF PEDIATRIC CANCER

Another considerable toll of childhood cancer on the family, one rarely addressed, is the way it drains incomes, by over 25 percent, on the average.

While your youngster is undergoing therapy, you will gladly spend your last penny to restore him to health. Not once did Craig or I so much as mention money. It was mutually understood that we would dip into the $25,000 in equity from the sale of our home in Storm Lake, money originally earmarked as a down payment on a new house in Worthington.

Two years later, when Jason's treatment began winding down, we decided that perhaps at last we should consider house hunting. What a rude awakening to discover we had nothing to buy a house with! As the two of us are still learning, the financial aftershocks of a child's cata-strophic illness rumble long after he is cured. To pay off our son's medical expenses, we had to borrow against a life-insurance policy as well as the full cash value of my husband's retirement pension, which we're slowly replenishing through monthly payments. I guess you could say we're indebted to the Mayo Clinic in more ways than one.

And here's the kicker: we had comprehensive health-care insurance. In this era of skyrocketing medical costs, until someone in your family is hospitalized with a serious illness, the fact that you're insured can lull you into a false sense of security. To begin with, over the months or years of treatment you run up myriad incidental—and uncovered—expenses: gasoline, lodging, food, parking, tolls, child care for other siblings. While you can usually negotiate a flexible payment schedule with the hospital, the motel cashier or the gas-station attendant de-mands cash or plastic on the spot. To prevent the liquid assets from drying up, Craig and I borrowed against our credit cards until they were charged to the limit. Then we refinanced them and started all over again.

More important, many parents mistakenly assume that once they've met their deductible (in our case, $2,000 a year), insurance covers X percent of all subsequent costs. Not quite. That is X share of *those fees the insurer deems reasonable,* a judgment occasionally subject to debate. For example, the Mayo Clinic charged $500 per X-ray procedure, which our insurance company contended was $200 higher than the state average. Therefore it reimbursed us 80 percent of only *$300,* or $240—a little less than half the actual cost. The remaining $260 came out of our pockets.

Contesting Disputed Claims

Midway through Jason's treatment Craig's employer switched insurers. Whereas the first company honored all claims without question, the second turned down a number of them, including a surgical procedure performed when Jason was nearly eleven. We referred to this earlier, but let me refresh your memory: the radiation sores inside his mouth were blocking his permanent teeth from coming in properly, so a Mayo Clinic surgeon had to "pull" them into position.

Our insurer refused to pay, declaring this *cosmetic* surgery. Cosmetic? On the cusp of adolescence, Jason still had his baby teeth. It was clearly a long-term complication of cancer therapy. The ensuing legal wrangling dragged on for two years. We submitted written testimonials justifying the surgery from Jason's physicians, other medical experts— everyone but the plumber, it seemed. What a headache.

In the interim the Mayo Clinic's billing department turned over our account to a collection agency, despite the fact that we'd always made every effort to clear our debt. Maybe each monthly payment wasn't as much as they would have liked, but I don't recall them returning any checks. Knowing that some patients renege completely on their obligations made it all the more irritating to receive harassing phone calls from the agency now and then.

We relate this not to editorialize against hospital-collection policies, simply to forewarn you. If you think that your family's problem entitles you to an exemption, think again. Medical centers are full of people with problems. That's their business. The person at the other end of the phone sees only a computer printout tallying your current liability, not your child's suffering. I realize that medical facilities are businesses and must be run accordingly, but it was a disillusioning experience nonetheless.

After my husband chewed out a collection agent over the phone one evening, we never heard from them again and could at least continue to whittle down our bill in peace. "Caught me on a bad day, she did," he says, not altogether regretfully. In the end the insurance company agreed to cover the surgery and reimburse the Mayo Clinic.

To reap the full benefits of your health insurance, we suggest the following:

• Study a current copy of your policy; know what is and is not covered.
• Refile any denied claims. Ask your physician to explain to the insurer why the service in question was medically necessary.

- Keep a running log of all medical expenses, including the type of service, the total charge, the amount paid by your insurer, the amount you paid, to whom, and the date and number of the check.
- Keep all medical records together.
- File claims for all covered costs. Don't be intimidated by the crush of paperwork involved. Twenty dollars here and there adds up.

If you feel your insurer has unfairly rejected a claim, the National Cancer Institute recommends registering a complaint in writing with the appropriate regulatory agency (see Appendix A). The address and telephone number of each is listed in the blue-pages section of your local white pages.

The hospital social worker or financial-aid counselor can advise you on writing the letter, provide sample letters to use as a guide, and obtain necessary documentation from your doctor. Your letter needn't be a scholarly essay. Describe the contested service, the grounds on which it was denied, and why you believe it meets the requirements for coverage. Make two copies, one for your files and one to send to the insurer. In your envelope to the regulatory agency enclose copies of any previous correspondence between you and your insurer as well as anything else you feel is germane.

Depending on the urgency of your case, these matters can take weeks or months to settle, but are definitely worth pursuing. According to Mayo Clinic social worker Ginny Rissmiller, "Some parents have written their congressmen about disputed insurance claims, and the congressmen have responded favorably."

Financial Aid

Pediatric-cancer patients may be eligible for financial assistance from government and volunteer agencies and pharmaceutical companies. Ask your hospital social worker or financial-aid counselor to contact those listed below or do so yourself *at once*. Much to our regret, by the time I discovered that we qualified for one state-administered program, Jason was in the final lap of treatment, and nothing was covered retroactively.

• ***Physically Handicapped Children's Program***   Also known as the Crippled Children's Program in some states, this program pro-

vides free medical, surgical, orthodontic, rehabilitative, and other related services to children with cancer and other chronic illnesses. Patients' families must meet certain age, medical, and financial
requirements, and these vary from state to state. To learn more, write
or call your county or state department of health, the address and
telephone number of which are listed in the blue-pages section of your
local white pages.

• *Supplemental Security Income (SSI)*   A federal program, SSI
provides financial aid to impoverished families with a disabled child.
Disabled is defined as "a physical or mental problem that keeps [the
patient] from working and is expected to last at least a year or to result
in death." The monthly amount for one youngster is $386 but may be
significantly more in states that supplement the federal check. For more
information, visit your local Social Security office or call toll-free (800)
772-1213 weekdays from seven A.M. to seven P.M. EST to arrange an
appointment with a Social Security representative.

• *The Leukemia Society of America's Patient-Aid Pro-
gram*   helps qualifying families defray the cost of leukemia, preleukemia, lymphoma, or multiple-myeloma treatment by paying up to
$750 a year of uncovered outpatient expenses, including drugs, blood
transfusions, and radiation. To learn if your child is eligible, call the
LSA information hotline (800-955-4LSA) or its New York City headquarters (212-573-8484).

• *The American Cancer Society*   lends the following items for
home health care: hospital beds, pillows, commodes, wheelchairs,
canes, wigs, dressings, prostheses, and various supplies for patients who
have undergone either an *ostomy* (surgically constructing an artificial
opening for eliminating bodily wastes, such as a colostomy) or a *laryngec-
tomy* (surgical procedure in which the voice box is partially or completely removed). Not all divisions provide the same services. Call your
regional ACS office at (800) ACS-2345 or its Atlanta national office
(404-320-3333).

• *Pharmaceutical-Company Patient-Assistance (Indigent
Patient) Programs*   According to the National Cancer Institute
eight pharmaceutical manufacturers presently supply chemotherapy
drugs free of charge to eligible patients. Your child's physician must
apply on your behalf. See Appendix A for names, addresses, and telephone numbers.

Suggestions on Conserving Money

All expenses related to essential medical treatment are tax-deductible. Save receipts for gas, food, taxi fares, lodging, and parking, and record in your journal car mileage to and from all doctors' appointments, therapy sessions, and pharmacies.

If you haven't in years past, hire an accountant to prepare your tax return. His knowledge of the deductions and benefits to which you're entitled should more than offset the fee.

When spending more than one night in a motel, find one with a kitchenette. Those times Jason and I couldn't get into Northland House, we stayed at an inexpensive—well, cheap—inn on the outskirts of Rochester. Cooking most of our own meals instead of eating out saved us a substantial sum, especially since several restaurants and coffee shops in the vicinity of the Mayo Clinic were unconscionably overpriced.

Carefully examine all hospital bills. Under the American Hospital Association's "Patient's Bill of Rights," you have the right to scrutinize and receive an explanation of your bill. Hospitals have been known to charge patients for procedures that were never performed, duplicate items on the bill, and exaggerate, or "upcode," treatment to resemble a more costly service. Clerical errors, such as accidentally transposing numbers so that a charge of $1,397 appears as $3,197, are distressingly common.

Craig and I confess to not having heeded this advice ourselves. When the medical bills began arriving, we were too absorbed in our son's needs to be bothered, stashing the reams of paper in a box. By the time I got around to leafing through them, it would have taken a battalion of accountants to decipher the cryptic abbreviations of procedures (some of which have multiple meanings) and to confirm every entry. I did the best I could, but I'm sure that some phantom charges or multiple billings slipped by me.

Ask your doctor about the cost of procedures beforehand. Several of the books we read about cancer suggested this, and we pass it on here with reservations. When a child's life is hanging in the balance, how many parents would refuse treatment because it was "too expensive"? I'd venture to guess very few.

"I could have cared less about money," recalls Craig. "I was going to take Jason any place he needed and get him whatever treatment he needed, no matter what it cost." Still, knowing a procedure should cost $200 will help you to spot the error should you be incorrectly billed $400 dollars.

CHAPTER TEN

SOURCES OF SUPPORT

Family and Friends • Support Groups • Faith

Contrary to popular mythology, childhood cancer doesn't strike only the resilient. And yet the majority of families afflicted exhibit a remarkable fortitude that frequently transcends their own expectations.

"I think if you asked any two parents if they could survive their child's cancer, they'd say no," observes Donna Betcher, Jason's favorite nurse. "But they would. You get strength, just as in any crisis.

"And you learn to rely on the people around you."

Craig and I derived much of our strength from those close to us and we remain eternally grateful to them for all their help and support. However, not every friend or relative has the same emotional capacity to handle a youngster's cancer. You may be surprised when support comes from those you'd least expect, and vice versa. You cannot predict people's reactions any more than you can foresee the outcome of the disease.

The weekend before Jason's diagnosis I visited my best friend, a woman I'd known since kindergarten, in my old hometown of Kingsley, Iowa. We shared the same birthday and for twenty-five years had spent every August 9 together celebrating. After my son got lymphoma, "Jane" vanished from my life. For the next five years there were no telephone calls, no get-well cards, nothing. I knew why too. Ten years earlier her younger brother had developed melanoma, and although treatment cured him, she simply couldn't face another life-threatening illness. Her fear of saying or doing the wrong thing paralyzed her.

My friend's behavior hurt and surprised me, but mostly I felt sorry for her. What did she think I wanted from her, some words that would magically ease our pain? She obviously had much greater expectations of herself than I did. An honest "I don't know what to say, but Jason is in my prayers" would have brought comfort enough.

Later that summer, when we were home from Jason's month of radiation treatments, someone knocked at the door. "I wonder who that could be?" I said to Craig. New in town, we barely knew a soul.

A woman about my age introduced herself as Colleen. "You don't know me, and I don't know you," she said. "But I heard what happened to your little boy, and it sounds to me like you could use a friend." With that she pushed open the screen door and stepped into our lives. Not surprisingly Colleen is still a very dear friend today.

A virtual stranger also came to Craig's rescue. One of his co-workers, a tall, gregarious Texan named Jerry, sensed he needed a friend and landed on our doorstep. "Hey, Craig, let's go out for a beer." "Hey, Craig, let's play some softball." Knowing how reserved my husband is, instead of calling first, Jerry just materialized, to offer a sympathetic ear. I don't know what we would have done without him and his wife, Darlene. That friendship too continues to flourish.

A youngster's potentially fatal illness leaves everyone feeling helpless. Still, most people feel they must say *something*, and that's when even the most sincere, well-meaning friends and family sometimes spout stale platitudes. Brace yourself for some of these jaw droppers:

"Well, we're all going to die someday."
"I guess it's just God's will."
"A boy down the block from us died of cancer."

And two that always left me speechless:

"At least you have three other kids." As if that would negate the loss.
"At least you and your husband are still young," implying that a new baby could replace Jason.

While there is no excuse for such seeming insensitivity, try not to take too much offense. In our culture death is usually a taboo subject. Just consider some of the many euphemisms we substitute for *dying:* "passing away," "departing," "expiring," death as "eternal sleep."

No wonder, then, that many people are uninformed about pediatric cancer and incapable of offering solace. It's extraordinary how many obsolete myths still circulate among basically intelligent adults: for instance, that a stricken child is doomed to die or that the disease is contagious. One idea for remedying people's lack of awareness is to order them extra copies of the free National Cancer Institute and American Cancer Society booklets recommended in Chapter Two and to suggest gently such people read them.

Children are nothing if not ingenuously honest and may drop callous remarks to your youngster. Once, as I was scrubbing the floor in the front hallway, I heard Jason, Adam, Tim, and some friends outside predicting their futures. "When I grow up," Jason declared, "I'm going to be a doctor at the Mayo Clinic."

"Unh-unh," interjected one boy. "My mom says you're gonna die before you grow up."

Grrrrrr. I had to stifle a roar, but Jason's indignant response brought a smile to my face.

"No sir, you don't know that! You could get hit by a car walking home from here and die before me! And I am too going to become a doctor."

"There but for the grace of God go I." I didn't have to be clairvoyant to sense that unspoken thought, the undercurrent of many an awkward conversation about Jason's condition. One child's cancer jars other parents into the grim realization that no family is invulnerable, and it can provoke some uneasy reactions. When answering concerned inquiries, I occasionally felt obligated to varnish the truth so that it seemed less threatening:

"How's Jason?"

"Oh, not too bad."

"Good!" You could almost hear the sigh of relief as they swiftly changed the subject.

For me this experience drew a line between acquaintances and true friends. A true friend, such as Colleen, flinched neither at the intimate details of our lives nor at my tears. "Is therapy helping Tim's stutter?" she would ask. "Does that medication seem to be controlling Jason's nausea?" Faking a cheerful façade for others when you really feel like crying is an immense strain. So I am thankful for friends like her, who allowed me to pour out my feelings freely.

Jason wasn't all we discussed. Far from it. At times cancer is the last thing you want to talk about. You need glimpses of a life beyond the disease, the life you're striving to regain. You also need to have an identity apart from Mother of a Young Cancer Patient. Believe me, to receive pitying looks or nominations for sainthood feels as isolating as total abandonment. You just want to be treated normally.

Relations and friends who appear to shy away at first haven't necessarily deserted you. They may want to help but don't want to impose, uncertain of your needs and state of mind. Another parent, for instance, may worry that it will upset you to be around her healthy children. Without a cue from you, how are others to know? If you haven't heard from someone close to you, break the ice and call them.

People often say, sincerely, "If there's anything I can do . . ." There is. Plenty. Sometimes we subconsciously push others away from us in times of crisis for fear of seeming needy, which we may associate as a sign of weakness. Accept friends' and relatives' offers and tell them what you need. This allows people to express feelings for you and your family that perhaps they cannot put into words. For parents of a young patient with siblings, or a single parent, nothing is more appreciated than help with managing the household. Let others:

- Invite siblings to their home for the day or for dinner
- Baby-sit
- Prepare freezable meals
- Spend the night with the patient, allowing you a sound night's sleep
- Run errands, to the drugstore, the grocery store, and so on
- Accompany you and your child to doctors' appointments
- Mow the grass, shovel snow
- Do the laundry, drop off and pick up dry cleaning

Several of our new neighbors in Worthington thoughtfully brought over casseroles, baked cookies for the kids, and took care of the lawn when we were away. Had we still been residing in Storm Lake, though, we could have depended upon an extensive support network. My husband and I found ourselves in the same position as many parents in today's increasingly mobile society, stranded in a strange town, with miles separating us from family and friends. A protracted medical crisis sure leaves you mourning the disintegration of the old-fashioned extended family.

Luckily Craig and I were able to rely on my parents, who exemplify our earlier statement about people exceeding your expectations. Without their physical, emotional, and financial support, our two-year odyssey would have exacted a far greater toll on everyone.

SUPPORT: FROM GRANDPARENTS

Grandmothers and grandfathers are often the forgotten grievers, and the family members hit hardest by a youngster's illness. Not only must they comfort the patient, but the patient's parents—their children—as well. Meanwhile who tends to *their* pain? Some cope by lapsing into denial, making it more difficult for them to lend support. In a survey where parents were asked to rank the people who aided them the most, the other spouse, friends, nurses and physicians, and other parents of ailing children all came before the grandparents.

Many mothers and fathers I've spoken to say they found it easier to tell their child she had cancer than to break the news to her grandparents. While you can perhaps burnish the facts for a young person ("Lots of people recover from cancer, honey"), Grandma and Grandpa understand the grave implications all too well.

Unquestionably, informing my parents and Craig's mother that their grandson had lymphoma was one of the hardest things I've ever done. Grandma Gaes was still grieving the death of her husband of thirty-six years. She and Fred had done everything together; one wouldn't even go to the grocery store without the other. "Mom lost thirty pounds over the next year," Craig remembers. "She took it pretty hard."

My elderly mother and father had also suffered a tragic loss. In 1966 my older brother, John, Jr., died in a car accident. He was just eighteen years old. As suddenly as he'd been snatched from us, our close-knit family unraveled. Dad anesthetized his sorrow with alcohol, while Mom quit work and grew highly protective of me and my three surviving brothers. It took years for everyone to regain their equilibrium. How would the two of them handle this latest adversity, one sure to dredge up awful memories? My mother, meanwhile, harbored the same concerns about me.

She remembers thinking, *"Oh, my God, now Geralyn is going to have to go through this.* I've often wondered which is the worst way to lose a child: like we did, where you go to the telephone and someone tells you, 'There's been a terrible accident; John is dead'? Or to watch your child die day by day? I don't think there's any question that to see him waste away is harder to bear.

"In the beginning," my mother confesses, "I wasn't sure if Geralyn could get through this."

From the day Jason was diagnosed, she and my father selflessly responded to our family's needs. First they turned over their business to someone else, then later that year sold their home in Storm Lake and moved into a townhouse just blocks away from our rented home on West Ninth Avenue. The two of them dropped everything to help run our household, cooking meals, washing clothes, and so on.

During the winter months, when the Minnesota weather turns unpredictable, Dad accompanied Jason and me to the Mayo Clinic. Some days he had to sit waiting in the main-floor lobby for upward of ten hours. "I must have read every newspaper that came into Rochester," he recalls with a chuckle, "but it was worth it to be able to be parked in front of the building with the car running and the heater on when Geralyn came out carrying Jason."

Having my parents available to look after the children afforded Craig and me the chance to get away once in a while. They'd call us up and say, "We don't have any plans for the weekend. How about if we watch the kids and you guys go to Minneapolis or Spirit Lake?" I felt secure with Mom taking care of Jason, which I could not have said about too many others. She knew, for example, to take her grandson's temperature if he seemed quiet, a signal that he didn't feel well.

Both my mother and my father were pillars of strength for us in a way they couldn't be for themselves twenty years earlier. In private, though, the stabs of anguish pierced their souls as deeply as my husband's and mine.

I'll never forget our first day at the Mayo Clinic. Dad had sat in on a question-and-answer session with Dr. Bringelsen, who explained the diagnosis and the proposed treatment. Afterward my father wrapped his arms around me and said confidently, "I really feel great having talked to the doctor. I just have a feeling that everything is going to be all right."

"That's great, Dad," I mumbled.

Dazed, I followed him out into the hall. My father, thinking I'd stayed behind in the conference room, leaned against a wall and began sobbing.

My mother remembers, "I'd go off in the car and cry by myself. Try to be strong. It was as if you had a weight on you all the time, like you could just break down at any moment."

Submerging their grief in the daily caretaking probably helped them both a great deal psychologically. Grandma Gaes, back in Storm Lake, might have suffered more, wondering and worrying. Although my husband's family love one another dearly, they were less involved. Everyone was still reeling from Fred Gaes's passing and struggling to keep his trucking business afloat. In effect they were in crisis too. It goes to show that not only do people respond differently to a child's cata-strophic illness, their capacity to respond hinges on events in their own lives.

SUPPORT: FROM SUPPORT GROUPS

Craig and I consider ourselves extremely lucky to have had my parents' unwavering support, for over the long haul people gradually return to their own affairs.

We've seen how the attendant stresses of childhood cancer continue to smolder long after the blaze has been contained. Even in the best of circumstances, where outside concern and caring remain constant, mothers and fathers may feel isolated and alone. A parent of a cancer patient is like an astronaut who's walked on the moon. She can vividly describe the experience to others, but unless they've actually done it themselves, it's difficult for them to truly understand.

Support groups, also known as self-help or peer-counseling groups, bring together people who share a common problem. I regret not having had the opportunity to join one for parents of children with cancer, as none existed within an hour's drive of Worthington. However, my casual discussions with other mothers and fathers at Rochester's Northland House fulfilled many of the same functions, so I believe I can attest to their effectiveness.

Isn't it depressing listening to a group of adults commiserate over their children's misfortunes? It can be, when, for example, someone's youngster suffers a setback. But you are more likely to hear inspiring success stories, a reflection of the steady progress made in cancer treatment. Consider that when the national support-group organization Candlelighters formed in 1970, only 20 percent of kids with cancer survived. Launched primarily to prepare parents for the inevitability of death, it and other parents' groups have become increasingly oriented toward continued life.

Groups can provide:

• ***Compassion, Understanding, Feedback.*** Hearing others confide their feelings validates your own. It was a relief for me to discover that my bouts of despondency weren't unique. Analyzing others' experiences can also help us identify our own problems and explore solutions.

• ***Education.*** Some of the more formal support groups engage outside speakers—medical professionals, psychologists, insurance-company representatives—to address issues of concern. But the most useful information often comes from the casual exchanges among group members, whose children are at different stages of the disease: postdiagnosis, completing therapy, in remission, newly relapsed, cured, dying.

• ***An Outlet for Raising Issues Outside the Realm of the Health-Care Team.*** Support groups give parents a forum for the emotional aspects of children's cancer that physicians and even social workers don't always address. No one at the Mayo Clinic ever asked, "How are you and your husband getting along? Any problems?" And if they had, I can't say I would have felt comfortable discussing it with them. In groups whose members have gradually established a bond of trust, intimate matters can be openly expressed in a nonjudgmental, empathetic atmosphere.

• ***Companionship.*** At a time when old friends may drop out of your life, support groups offer an opportunity for forming new friendships.

• ***A Network of Practical Support.*** Members can arrange to baby-sit for one another, carpool to doctors' appointments, run errands, raise money for medical expenses, and so forth.

Support groups for young patients and for their siblings have also sprung up around the country. They may be as formal or informal as the members desire. Some are designed purely as discussion groups, while others promote education by featuring guest speakers and films and maintaining lending libraries of relevant books and articles.

The success or failure depends on the chemistry among the participants and the competence of the group coordinator-discussion leader. This *facilitator* may be a psychiatric nurse, a social worker, a psychotherapist, a clergyman, or the parent of a child with cancer. Ideally he or she will foster constructive dialogues that offer mutual support and encouragement, as well as realistic advice and coping strategies.

FINDING A SUPPORT GROUP

• *The Candlelighters Childhood Cancer Foundation*   (1312 18th Street, N.W., Suite 200, Washington, D.C. 20036, 800-366-2223; 202-659-5136 in Washington, D.C.) is an international nonprofit network of over three hundred support groups, mainly for parents but also for brothers and sisters, patients, and whole families.

Local Candlelighters groups sponsor crisis phone lines, buddy systems, parent-to-parent contacts, professional counseling, family social functions, and blood banks. They additionally offer such services as baby-sitting, transportation, waiting-room aides, hospital-patient visits, donating wigs and clothing to families, and setting up residences for families of children receiving therapy away from home. Interested family members may receive the Foundation's quarterly newsletter and youth newsletter free of charge.

• *Make Today Count*   (P.O. Box 6063, Kansas City, Kansas 66106, 913-362-2866). This nonprofit national self-help organization for patients with a life-threatening disease and their families was formed in 1975 by the late Orville Kelly, a midwestern newspaperman stricken with lymphoma. Approximately seventy local MTC groups are scattered across the United States, providing many of the same services as the Candlelighters.

• *The American Cancer Society*   (regional offices, 800-ACS-

2345; national office, 1599 Clifton Road, N.E., Atlanta, Georgia 30329, 404-320-3333) administers two free programs: CanSurmount pairs cancer patients with trained volunteers who either have or have had cancer, for one-to-one communication and support. Likewise family members are matched with other parents and siblings of young people with the disease.

I Can Cope, open to patients and family members, is an education program on living with cancer. Over the course of eight two-hour weekly sessions, physicians, nurses, social workers, and other health-care professionals impart practical information and answer questions about coping with the physical and emotional side effects of cancer treatment.

• *The Leukemia Society of America* (733 Third Avenue, New York, New York 10017, 800-955-4LSA, 212-573-8484) operates thirty-two groups nationally for parents, siblings, patients, and anyone else who wants to attend. All are led by professionals with experience in oncology, such as physicians, nurses, social workers, and marriage and family therapists.

• In addition to national organizations, there are regional and local programs throughout the country. For instance, Cancer Care, a non-profit social-services agency, serves the tristate New York–New Jersey–Connecticut area, while Missouri and Kansas residents have access to a variety of support groups through the R. A. Bloch Cancer Support Center in Kansas City, Missouri. To learn of regional and local self-help groups in your vicinity, call the Cancer Information Service (800-4-CANCER), the American Cancer Society (regional offices, 800-ACS-2345; national office, 404-320-3333), or ask your hospital social worker.

• Most cancer centers conduct their own in-house support groups. Unfortunately since we lived so far from the Mayo Clinic, I was able to take part only once or twice, when Jason was hospitalized. Should you feel it necessary, many hospitals also offer individual and family counseling with on-staff or on-call therapists, psychologists, or psychiatrists who specialize in working with family members touched by cancer. The social worker can also refer you to mental-health services provided by your county health department.

• If there are no groups near your home, you may want to consider starting your own, either under the aegis of a national organization such as the Candlelighters or through a local medical center. All you need are two or three interested parties. We'd suggest finding a nurse, social worker, or some other oncology professional to volunteer as a consultant.

While I personally gained a great deal from conversing with other parents, support groups are not for everyone. You may feel that this disease consumes enough of your time and energy as it is. Or that you're not comfortable sharing your personal life with strangers. Or, like my husband, you may find all the talk about cancer discouraging. Then again, you may simply decide you enjoy all the support you need from family and friends. Certainly no one should participate in a group if he is not ready emotionally; it's a good idea to sort out your feelings in private first.

But don't deny yourself support because you equate seeking help with some weakness or inadequacy on your part. Cancer *is* overwhelming; avail yourself of the support systems at your disposal. Remember that your child needs you to be there for him. Sometimes the best way to ensure that is to have someone there for you.

SUPPORT: FROM FAITH

For those who choose to believe in a higher power, nothing tests their faith more rigorously than a youngster's potentially fatal illness. It can disrupt most basic beliefs about the way and order of the world and can raise troubling doubts. How could this happen to an innocent child? What sort of God would impose such suffering?

Those were the very questions Craig asked himself, and the answers he received then were not reassuring. If you recall, the night that Jason was diagnosed with lymphoma, my mother suggested we all repair to the Saint Marys Hospital chapel and pray. "You go ahead and pray," was my husband's blunt reply. "I'm all done praying."

Craig, raised in the Lutheran Church, converted to Catholicism for our wedding. It wasn't an issue between us or our families. We merely decided we should be one or the other, and I'd been a practicing Catholic from the time I was a little girl. "Geralyn's faith was a bigger part of her life," Craig says matter-of-factly. "I didn't really have strong feelings about it."

Beginning that night at Saint Marys, however, and for a long time afterward Craig's bitterness threatened to consume him. "At the time," he remembers, "I felt, *First he took my dad, and now he wants to take my little boy. Why would you want to kneel down in front of a God like that?*" He stopped going to mass, believing that the Lord had deserted him.

"Craig took it awful," says Grandma Gaes, "because he already missed his father. He said to me, 'Why is God punishing me like this?' I told him, 'Craig, don't feel that way. God doesn't punish people by giving their little boys cancer. He's probably making us stronger through this.' I tried to give him a little strength; that's all I could do. 'Your dad's up above,' I said. 'He'll help us through.' I always believed that."

Concerned about Craig, I visited our priest when we came home to Worthington in early July. "We don't really know anyone in town," I explained. "My husband needs a friend, somebody to talk to." The priest nodded thoughtfully and said he'd be in touch soon.

I never heard from him again. It was shortly after this that Craig's co-worker, Jerry, burst into our lives, assuming the supportive role I'd expected the clergy to play. Ironically I discovered more Christ-like qualities in this rough-talking but tenderhearted cowboy than I did in much of the church hierarchy in whom I'd invested so much faith. Again, it demonstrates that your anticipated sources of comfort don't always deliver, not even the professed experts we think we can turn to. And why should they? It's very likely that priest had never encountered a child with cancer before. Perhaps, like so many others, he didn't know how to respond either.

Sometimes I'd get upset when Craig wouldn't attend Sunday-morning mass, feeling it set a bad example for the kids. But then I'd think, *Can you ask someone to change his values if that's what he truly believes?* For my husband to become a hypocrite wouldn't have provided such a shining example either.

In the end it took Jason to help restore his father's faith. Throughout his illness "I prayed to God a lot," says our son. "I think it helped me get through having cancer." During tests he nervously used to finger the silver crucifix that dangled from his neck, a gift from his uncle Francis. While Jason and I were out shopping one day, he spotted a small plaque containing a parable he felt would hold special meaning for his father:

Footprints in the Sand

One night a man had a dream. He dreamed he was walking along the beach with the Lord. Across the sky flashed scenes from his life. For each scene, he noticed two sets of footprints in the sand; one belonging to him, and the other to the Lord.

When the last scene of his life flashed before him, he looked back at the footprints in the sand. He noticed that many times along the path of his life there was only one set of footprints. He also noticed that it happened at the very lowest and saddest times in his life.

This really bothered him, and he questioned the Lord about it. "Lord, you said that once I decided to follow you, you'd walk with me all the way. But I have noticed that during the most troublesome times in my life there is only one set of footprints. I don't understand why when I needed you most you would leave me."

The Lord said, "My precious, precious child, I love you, and I would never leave you. During your times of trial and suffering, when you see only one set of footprints, it was then that I carried you."

—Author unknown

Craig has kept that plaque on his nightstand ever since. "I don't know that I'm fully back with the church yet," he says. But a few summers after Jason got well, we all went to see the movie *Ghost*, about a murder victim whose soul lingers to protect his lover still here on earth. "You know," Craig remarked on our way out of the theater, "I wonder if that's what Dad did when Jason got sick: watch over him until he was sure everything would be okay."

Although we reacted differently in the long run, I certainly understood Craig's anger. When something like this happens, it's got to be somebody's fault, so who else do you blame it on but God? Who else could have controlled the series of events that resulted in Jason's cancer? It nearly shattered my faith, too, at first.

My son would ask me, "Why did Jesus do this to me? Why did he pick me?" And I had no reply, because I was struggling with that question myself. I suppose we all accept that bad things happen to good people, but when it's *your child* . . . Well, as a Christian who believed in a loving, merciful God, I just could not conceive of a heavenly plan that included the suffering and possible death of my six-year-old.

Jason's cancer violently shook the foundation of my religion. Which made me feel *terrible,* to be at odds with God. I sometimes wonder what would have happened had he not survived. It's kind of scary. Your faith isn't always as steadfast as you think it is.

Instead I chose to believe that the Lord would help me if I asked him. For me, the Scriptures were the only place where I could find any guarantee that Jason would live. The doctors could tell us, "We'll try," "We'll do the best we can." But the God I worship says, "Ask and it shall be given to you." And so I asked every night.

CHAPTER ELEVEN

BACK TO SCHOOL

Preparing Faculty and Classmates • Classroom
Presentations • A Cancer Patient's Special Needs

Ask our son if he likes school, and he replies brightly, "Sure!" Then
comes the qualifier: "When the bell rings, I start hating it." Ah, yes, if
it weren't for those annoying classes. We're presently investigating
colleges that offer majors in lunch and recess, Jason's two favorite
subjects.

Whatever their prior attitudes toward school, most young patients
are eager to return, if not for the education, then to be with their pals
again. Jason, no exception, was excited to enter first grade in late
August. To him it represented the end of that awful summer and a
partial return to normalcy. "School was a place where I didn't have to
worry about anything," he says. "Where I could just be myself, not 'the
little sick boy.'"

PREPARING CLASSMATES

Starting school was going to be an important step for my son, and I hoped to make the transition as smooth as possible. Several books and pamphlets I read all recommended having the patient's teacher openly discuss his disease with his classmates, for kids enlightened as to the causes and consequences of cancer are generally less fearful of an ill youngster. Furthermore students frequently take their behavioral cues from authority figures. A teacher who appears at ease with the subject is more likely to convey that sensibility to her class than one who seems uncomfortable talking about it.

I arranged a conference with the principal of the boys' parochial school, at which I outlined the events of the past three months, Jason's special needs, the symptoms he might exhibit, the unpredictability of his treatment schedule, and so on. When I suggested that the school nurse or someone else knowledgeable about pediatric cancer briefly speak to his class the first day of school, the principal shook her head.

"I don't think that'd be a good idea," she said. "Let's not make an issue of Jason's sickness unless we have to. If a problem comes up, we'll address it then."

My heart told me this was a formula for disaster. Did she truly believe the other kids weren't going to notice Jason's bald head and bloated face? His periodic drowsy spells? But, somewhat intimidated, I deferred to her judgment. *She's a professional when it comes to kids,* I thought. *I guess she knows what's best.*

"The first morning of school," Jason recalls, "I walked into the classroom, and everyone just kind of stared at me. All the kids' mouths fell to the floor. I could hear some of them laughing, so I felt embarrassed. At recess lots of kids made fun of me."

Compounding matters, we'd moved to Worthington with only six weeks left in the previous school year. For all intents Jason was still the New Kid, which in itself branded him an outsider. When even the handful of boys he'd befriended in kindergarten acted standoffish as well, I knew we had a serious problem on our hands.

My immediate impulse was to march back to the principal's office—not to mention my desire to throttle the little bullies taunting my sick child. But I refrained, knowing that children usually prefer to settle disputes themselves, without parental interference. At home Jason remained tight-lipped about what was going on, although his watchful brother, Adam, kept me apprised of teasing and other minor incidents. Once in a while Jason would bemoan that nobody picked him for kickball or wanted him as their math partner. As I'm sure other parents will understand, it was painful to witness his misery.

One day that fall while Jason convalesced at home from surgery, I impulsively dropped in on the principal. The situation was clearly being mishandled, and it was up to me to act as my son's advocate. Politely but firmly I told her, "The other kids don't know what's the matter with Jason and treat him like a leper. I think somebody should talk to the class."

This time the principal agreed. "I'd be happy to talk to the children. But I don't know that much about cancer," she admitted.

"Well, *I'd* talk to them," I offered.

"Then why don't we do that right now?"

Next thing I knew, I was explaining cancer to a roomful of curious first-graders. When I finished, hands shot up in the air: "How did Jason get cancer?" they wanted to know. "Can we get it from him?" "Why does he look so funny?" "How come he misses so many days of school?" "Will Jason get better?" "Is he going to die?"

No one knew how or why Jason got cancer, I replied, but it wasn't contagious like a cold or the measles. In simple terms I described how the treatment to get rid of it made Jason's hair fall out, and so on. As for questions about his prognosis, I told the children that there were many different kinds of cancer. "Some people do die," I said, "but Jason's doctors are working very hard to make him better."

As I spoke, the fear melted from their faces. The majority of the children didn't mean to hurt Jason's feelings, they simply did not understand why this little boy looked so odd. And, regrettably, the school's reluctance to acknowledge candidly Jason's obvious differences only reinforced their suspicions that he was someone to avoid.

"With a cancer diagnosis many people still believe that the child is going to die," says Mayo Clinic pediatric-oncology social worker Ginny Rissmiller, who assists parents with their youngster's school reentry. "By not telling Jason's peers anything, the school was assuming the worst, and the secretive approach backfired.

"When children are educated about a classmate's cancer," she emphasizes, "you see more openness."

There are a number of other ways for children to learn about a classmate's illness. The teacher might make cancer the topic for a health- or science-class report. Treatment centers and organizations such as the American Cancer Society and the Candlelighters can often send a nurse or other qualified person to speak.

But perhaps the most effective method is to let the young person get up in front of the class and talk about his condition. Later that year Jason wrote and read aloud a paper on Burkitt's lymphoma. The students saw him not as a patient but as a kid just like them, one who happened to be living with a disease.

My informal talk to Jason's class made all the difference in the world. His first day back at school from surgery, the other boys and girls crowded around him and said with newfound respect and sympathy, "Wow, we didn't know you were going through all that. Now we know what's the matter with you."

"Guess what!" he announced happily that night at dinner. "I got picked second in kickball!" He never felt like an outcast again. And the one bully who continued to pick on him, calling Jason "Baldy," was soon silenced by big-brother Adam with a little frontier—make that schoolyard—justice.

For Jason that was the last of the teasing. Some young patients, however, face a much harder time. Teachers may be reluctant to step in, out of concern that the other children will perceive their intervention as favoritism. Chronic teasing, even if meant in fun, can make a youngster feel so self-conscious that he avoids school altogether. Long before that happens, a teacher should confront the transgressor and ascertain what's behind his behavior. Is he frightened of the young person with cancer? Resentful of the attention he gets? Just naturally aggressive? Through discussion and role-playing, teachers can help teasing children understand their reactions and correct the problem.

PREPARING TEACHERS
FOR THE RETURNING CHILD

Our experience was a textbook example of how *not* to have a child with cancer return to school. My first mistake was in assuming that faculty members would know how to manage the situation. As I discovered, this is an issue they rarely, if ever, encounter. Teachers, like students, need to be educated about this disease.

As soon as possible after a cancer diagnosis, someone should contact the child's principal, teacher(s), school nurse, and school psychologist, alerting them to the youngster's condition and explaining the impact this will have on his school attendance and classroom participation. Your hospital social worker can assume this ongoing responsibility, keeping school personnel abreast of developments regarding the patient's health and education throughout treatment. Or you may wish to handle it yourself.

Next, the school nurse should obtain from your child's physician all pertinent releases and medical records. Older children, especially teenagers, may be reluctant to let others know of their illness, fearing they'll be shunned or teased. Explain to your child that when everyone has accurate information, they will be much less likely to gossip or treat him differently.

Ask one or more members of your child's medical team, perhaps the primary physician and the social worker, to collaborate on a letter to be circulated among school personnel. It should address:

- The treatment's effect on the young person's attendance. Will she be attending full days, or are partial days more realistic?
- How she appears to be coping emotionally with her disease.
- Her feelings about returning to school.
- Any changes in her physical appearance due to the disease or therapy.
- How medications may affect her classroom performance.
- Anticipated physical reactions to medication.
- Special arrangements for transportation to and from school, if necessary.
- Whether or not she can participate in physical-education class. If so, what activities are restricted or prohibited?

• Special health needs, such as a rest period, access to a teachers' rest room, mid-morning snacks.

Once faculty members have had an opportunity to read the letter, request a conference to include teachers, administrators, counselors, the school nurse and/or psychologist, and anyone else involved with your child's return to school. This is a good time for everyone to agree on a key contact at the school who will relay information to the others.

Your role at this meeting is to establish a rapport with the faculty and to create the most supportive environment for your child. Use this time to:

• Encourage understanding of the myriad physical, emotional, and social challenges the patient faces. Bring along pamphlets and other literature, hot-line numbers, and perhaps a list of suggested books. Craig and I highly recommend the booklets "Back to School: A Handbook for Teachers of Children with Cancer," from the American Cancer Society (800-ACS-2345), and "Students with Cancer: A Resource for the Educator," from the National Cancer Institute (800-4-CANCER). Both are free and can be ordered in bulk.
• Formulate disciplinary guidelines. Teachers don't always know what limits to set for a child with cancer. While some may bend the rules out of pity, others may feel compelled to show other students that the patient's illness doesn't entitle him to special treatment. Whatever boundaries apply to other children should apply to yours too. Allowances beyond your youngster's physical and emotional needs could very easily arouse resentment. Faculty should regard this crisis as temporary and understand that the young person's normal social and emotional development must not be compromised at this crucial time.
• Plan a realistic academic schedule and goals that take into account your child's projected attendance yet satisfy course requirements. These may need periodic revision.

Special-Education Programs and Services

For a year and a half Jason missed an average of three school days every two weeks. I lobbied his teachers and administrators for special tutoring, summer school, anything to get him caught up, but they were unresponsive. Their attitude seemed to be, "He's going to die anyway, so why bother?"

This had a profound impact on Jason. When we finally transferred him and Tim to a public school following fourth grade, he read at a second-grade level. The public school had better resources and, perhaps more importantly, a willingness to work with Jason. A year later my son's reading skills were up to par.

Some children with cancer suffer learning disabilities, one of the potential long-term consequences covered in detail in Chapter Fourteen. Those who otherwise reason well and think clearly may have difficulty with tasks that require quick mental processing and memory. While these problems might initially appear developmental in nature, in fact they may indicate a real loss of intellectual ability.

Youngsters with brain tumors or who have received cranial radiation are especially at risk. Often problems with processing, memory, vision, walking, socialization, and self-image are readily apparent, and the school can provide the appropriate services. Be aware, however, that too often these changes are so subtle, they elude detection.

Every seriously ill or handicapped child has special rights to education under Public Law 94-142, known as the Education of All Handicapped Act. It requires every state to make available free and suitable education to *all* handicapped children between ages three and twenty-one.

Public Law 94-142 ensures the following services:

- Supplementary tutoring in specific subjects
- Instruction at home or in the hospital any time your child is absent for more than a few days
- Specialized physical education
- Makeup exams
- Waiver of automatic school-absence penalties
- Reorganization of class schedule
- Special equipment
- Counseling for school-related problems

Because the language of the law is somewhat vague, compliance varies from state to state. Not all school districts routinely offer special services, even when they know a child needs them. This is one area where you may have to be assertive and persistent. Just remember, the law is on your side.

Under the law the school must design an *Individual Education Plan,* or IEP, for each child. Request from your youngster's school, in writing, an assessment of his intellectual and emotional development and consideration of placement in a special-education program. Do this as soon after diagnosis as possible, so that testing can be complete and your child's special program in place if needed. In fact it's not a bad idea to request an IEP even if your child seems to be doing well attending regular classes. Circumstances may change, and you want to be prepared.

Generally every child with cancer should have a thorough educational and psychological evaluation, especially if he is starting kindergarten or first grade or is at high risk for learning disabilities.

Once the IEP evaluation is complete, the school district has a deadline (varying from state to state) in which to call a meeting. Parents are required to attend, preferably accompanied by a health-care professional familiar with the patient's case. The purpose of the meeting is to devise a concrete plan for the child's education, taking into consideration the following:

- Long- and short-term goals during the IEP term
- The child's current functioning level (social, behavioral, physical, academic) compared with that of other children the same age
- Possible settings (regular classes plus special services; use of a resource room for part of the day; special-education class for all or most of the day) and special services needed for him to function in each
- Appropriate physical and vocational education

The school district will appoint a case manager, or liaison (often a special-education teacher), responsible for monitoring your child's progress.

Handling Physical Challenges

School personnel should fully understand your child's health needs and how to respond to potential problems. For example, the school nurse must know what to do in case of bleeding, vomiting, fainting, and so on.

Ask your doctor to write a letter outlining proper procedures. Warn everyone not to administer *any* drug—not even aspirin, which could induce uncontrollable bleeding—without your and/or your child's doctor's permission. Many schools offer routine immunizations, and these, too, are strictly forbidden without your doctor's approval. In addition supply the faculty with the phone numbers of the nearest hospital, your child's physician, and you and your spouse.

Even a child who feels well enough to attend school may need extra help or attention with one or several of the physical problems listed below. By addressing and finding solutions to these early on, you'll make your youngster's school experience more enjoyable and productive.

• *Weakness, Impaired Coordination from Chemotherapy, or Amputation.* Some children might need extra time to get from class to class. If a multistory school building has an elevator, request permission for your child to use it when necessary.

• *General Fatigue.* Jason often had to nap at his desk or in the nurse's office. Because his teacher and I had agreed beforehand that he could rest at his own discretion, my son didn't even have to raise his hand for permission to leave the classroom. Those times when he was simply too exhausted to continue, I'd be called to take him home.

• *Nausea and Vomiting.* Jason carried with him at all times a covered plastic container that we dubbed his barf can. My son usually grew nauseous around noontime, when cafeteria aromas wafted through the halls. It's impossible to predict just what might set off nausea, but a youngster who is prepared feels less anxious. Include in his bookbag or lunchbox a travel toothbrush, toothpaste, a miniature bottle of mouthwash, and breath mints.

• *Need to Use Special Rest-Room Facilities.* If your child requires a waste-collecting device, she may feel self-conscious about using the girls' room. Arrange for her to be allowed into a faculty rest room or the nurse's office rest room. You might also consider this if your youngster experiences frequent nausea, diarrhea, or other problems she finds embarrassing.

• *Exposure to Disease.* Of particular concern to parents of a young cancer patient is *chicken pox,* a highly contagious virus that in most healthy children runs its course without complication. But to a child with a compromised immune system, it can be life-threatening.

Theoretically anyone who has already had chicken pox is immune to future outbreaks. However, in young people undergoing chemotherapy the chicken pox virus may manifest as the blistery skin rash *shingles*. If you suspect your child has been exposed to chicken pox, or should a suspicious rash erupt, notify the doctor immediately.

Scientists have yet to develop a chicken-pox vaccine. Therefore only the vigilance of school personnel and other parents can protect your youngster. Teachers should keep the ill child *and his siblings* away from anyone with chicken pox and notify you of all cases immediately.

A cancer patient exposed to chicken pox will usually not break out in the telltale sores for ten to twenty-one days. However, one to five days before the onset of symptoms, he is highly contagious.

During Jason's second year in grade school a little girl who sat next to him in class came down with chicken pox. Because everyone knew to be on the lookout, his teacher phoned me immediately. Jason's doctor injected him with *zoster immune globulin*, acronymed ZIG. If administered within seventy-two hours, ZIG and another medication, *zoster immune plasma* (ZIP), can thwart or at least weaken the still-incubating virus. Much to my relief, Jason never did come down with the disease.

To alert other parents to the danger chicken pox poses to a cancer patient, the American Cancer Society suggests distributing copies of the following sample letter to faculty and each student's parents:

> Dear Parents and School Staff,
> My (daughter/son) is a member of this year's (first, second, etc.) grade class. Recently (she/he) was diagnosed as having cancer. Currently (she/he) is in remission from cancer and is doing well, and we expect (her/him) to continue to be well.
>
> I am writing this letter for two reasons. The first is to make you aware of (her/his) disease and to reassure you that cancer is *not contagious*. The second is to ask for your help.
>
> My (daughter's/son's) cancer is being controlled by chemotherapy, which kills the cancer cells in the blood but also kills some of the normal cells. When the normal cells die, there can be a problem of lowered immunity, which means it is more difficult to fight infection, especially viral infections such as chicken pox.

If my (daughter/son) were to contract these illnesses, it could be very serious. Therefore I need to know if your child is exposed to or has contracted chicken pox. If I know that my child has been exposed, (she/he) can take medicine to lessen the effects.

Please feel free to ask me any questions. Thank you for your help.

Sincerely,

_____

Name

_____

Phone Number

_____

School Phone Number

In addition to chicken pox, your child's doctor may be concerned about his exposure to other diseases, such as rubella. If so, include them in your letter.

PRESCHOOL AND NURSERY SCHOOL

Children of preschool or nursery-school age can benefit immensely from participation in a class. For one thing it gives you and your youngster a break. His few hours a day out of the house affords you extra time to spend with siblings, your spouse, friends, or neighbors; run errands; take an exercise class; or simply relax and recharge.

Preschool or nursery-school classes help children develop social and developmental skills. Playing with other kids, making new friends, and having fun teaches them age-appropriate abilities needed for success in kindergarten. Seriously ill children rarely get to play as much as others, or if they do, their activities are restricted. While the abilities a child masters through play may seem basic, youngsters who miss out on these experiences may fall behind their classmates once they start school. If necessary, your child's teacher can advise you on developing these skills at home or whenever illness keeps him out of class.

The preschool or nursery-school experience also teaches a child independence. Once your youngster is confident that his stay in class is temporary and that you will be there for him at the end of the day, he'll have an easier time tolerating your short absences in other situations.

KEEPING YOUNG PATIENTS
FEELING CONNECTED

Your child's teacher can ensure that he feels part of his class even when confined at home or in the hospital. Prolonged absences should be discussed openly with the other students, who, if uninformed, may grow anxious and imagine the worst. The teacher can set aside class time for writing letters and making cards. She might also coordinate hospital or home visits from classmates, if allowed, and encourage telephone calls.

Your youngster's experiences and accomplishments in school can be a source of fulfillment and happiness during an otherwise difficult time. School provides children with not only academic training but also opportunities to develop as full human beings, through friendship, activities, and achievement.

CHAPTER TWELVE

THE MOMENT OF TRUTH

Unproven Cancer Treatments • Questions to Ask the Doctor
and the Anesthesiologist • Preoperative Procedures

No sooner had our son returned to school than the doctors told us he would have to undergo major surgery. Chemotherapy had dissolved the cancerous growths on Jason's kidneys and dramatically shrunk the tumor in his abdomen from ten inches down to two, but then it ceased to work further. "He might be developing an immunity to the drugs," one of his physicians warned. If so, and the malignancy commenced growing again, there would be no way to stop it. The doctors felt they had no choice but to remove the stubborn fragment surgically.

Anytime there's a medical setback, parents may be inclined to vent anger at their child's physicians for having "failed." I can recall one mother who reacted this way, lashing out at the doctors as if they had caused her daughter's relapse. The little girl, afflicted with bone cancer, had lost a leg. Her oncologists recommended no further therapy, apparently confident that the amputation had removed all cancer. Sometime later, however, the disease materialized in the child's lungs. Her mother charged that the medical team should have been more aggressive and followed the surgery with chemotherapy as a precaution. "I shouldn't have listened to them; I should have gone somewhere else," she said bitterly. Though I never felt that way myself, I can understand her frustration and need to lay blame somewhere.

UNPROVEN CANCER TREATMENTS

Any obstacle on the path to recovery leaves a young cancer patient's mother and father dangerously vulnerable to the fantastic claims of scientifically unproven cures. Faced with the possibility of their child's death, they will grasp at any chance. Unfortunately, alternative therapies do not cure cancer. While parents and patients reach for those branches of promise, the clock is ticking, and time that could be spent on a more effective, proven treatment is squandered.

You've no doubt read or heard about some of these unconventional regimens, such as nutritional therapy, which includes repeated coffee enemas, and vitamin therapy. Tests conducted by the medical establishment demonstrate conclusively that neither is effective against cancer. In fact both are potentially dangerous. The low-protein, low-calorie macrobiotic diet prescribed by some proponents can literally starve a person to death, while excessive doses of vitamins may accumulate in the body and produce toxic side effects.

Probably the most publicized unorthodox cancer remedy of recent years was *laetrile*, also known as vitamin B_{17}. Derived mainly from apricots and almonds, laetrile is comprised primarily of the extremely poisonous substance amygdalin, which the body converts to cyanide. Its developers, a German-immigrant physician and his doctor son, were not at all charlatans but genuinely believed they were onto a promising cure.

Word of the new wonder drug sent tens of thousands of patients scurrying to Mexico and other foreign countries to receive it, for laetrile is illegal in approximately half the fifty states. Beginning in 1957 cancer researchers tested the substance extensively in animals, revealing no evidence that it killed tumors. Despite these findings, the claims for laetrile escalated, and so in 1981 the federal government dispensed it to human volunteers in a clinical trial.

According to the National Cancer Institute safety review board report issued the following year, laetrile proved completely ineffective in shrinking malignancies, extending survival time, or relieving symptoms of the disease. At the same time laetrile is not harmless, having caused fatal and near-fatal cyanide poisoning even when taken in recommended doses. Several of those victims were children.

Along with some two dozen other dubious therapies, laetrile is included on a list of unproven methods of cancer management published by the American Cancer Society. If you are considering alternative treatment for your child, we urge you to call the ACS (800-ACS-2345 or 404-320-3333) for a free detailed statement on any or all of the following:

- Dr. Hariton-Tzannis Alivizatos's Greek Cancer Cure
- Antineoplastons
- Vlastimil (Milan) Brych
- Chaparral tea
- Contreras Methods
- Dimethyl Sulfoxide (DMSO)
- Electronic devices
- Gerson Method
- Hoxsey Method
- Immuno-Augmentative Therapy of Lawrence Burton, Ph.D., Bahamas
- Iscador
- Laetrile
- Live Cell Therapy
- Livingston-Wheeler Therapy
- Macrobiotic diets for the treatment of cancer
- Metabolic Cancer Therapy of Harold W. Manner, Ph.D.
- Nutritional and Metabolic Cancer Therapy of William D. Kelley
- Psychic surgery
- Revici Method
- O. Carl Simonton, M.D.

For the opposing viewpoint, you might wish to contact the following nonprofit educational organizations, which support and publish free literature about unorthodox holistic therapies:

- Foundation for Advancement in Cancer Therapies (FACT), P.O. Box 1242, Old Chelsea Station, New York, New York 10113, (212) 741-2790

• International Association of Cancer Victors and Friends (IACVF), 7740 West Manchester Avenue, Suite 110, Playa del Rey, California 90293, (213) 822-5032

Another agency, CanHelp, charges a fee to review a patient's medical records, consult with a worldwide network of medical advisers, and prepare a report on the appropriate treatment options. Its address and telephone number are 3111 Paradise Bay Road, Port Ludlow, Washington 98365, (206) 437-2291.

We don't feel it is our place to discourage parents from researching other forms of treatment for their child. But having read the literature of these and other groups, I have to say their inflammatory language and grand-conspiracy theories make me uneasy. They refer to the National Cancer Institute, the American Cancer Society, and other arms of the medical mainstream with such derisive terms as "known enemies of alternative cancer therapies" and "the Cancer Church," and accuse them of greedily suppressing public awareness of unorthodox methods. Or, in other words, crushing the competition.

The IACVF's quarterly newsletter claimed, "The NCI has steadfastly refused to conduct formal clinical trials into promising alternative cancer therapies, repeatedly seeking to discredit those physicians and scientists who have pursued independent and innovative avenues of research." The facts, however, repudiate that charge.

As mentioned earlier, the U.S. government thoroughly investigated laetrile. Next consider the case of Dr. Hariton-Tzannis Alivizatos's Greek Cancer Cure, offered in Athens, Greece, and Tijuana, Mexico, site of several cancer clinics. Dr. Alivizatos, a Greek microbiologist, claims to have "cured" an incredible 80 to 86 percent of his patients suffering from advanced cancer by injecting them with a serum six times daily for thirty days.

After the doctor refused to divulge the composition of this serum, Greek authorities suspended his medical license for two years. Additionally Dr. Alivizatos maintains no records on the clients he treats—at $2,000 per person, including the stay in Athens—and refuses to provide evidence of his findings for independent scientific review. Five times between 1981 and 1989 the American Cancer Society and the National Cancer Institute formally requested documentation regarding the Greek Cancer Cure, but received only one response: a letter from Dr. Alivizatos himself stating he had nothing to submit.

Despite Dr. Alivizatos's lack of supporting documentation, the IACVF has entered this therapy in its list of alternative and adjunctive treatment centers. The American Cancer Society strongly urges patients not to seek treatment based on the recommendations of the IACVF, which, it states, appears to neither research, analyze, nor evaluate the effectiveness and safety of the treatment methods it promotes.

Interestingly, that same list bears the curious disclaimer, "The IACVF does not recommend or endorse in this instance, nor does it assume any responsibility." The association advises anyone contemplating alternative treatment "to investigate carefully the doctor, the product and the price before deciding on a course of action," but fails to explain just how a layperson would go about doing this. What recourse does he have outside of reading the treatment centers' own self-serving promotional literature?

Are all purveyors of unproven cancer-control methods hucksters? No, not all. But Dr. Smithson, expressing the predominant viewpoint among physicians associated with recognized medical institutions, believes the majority are. "I personally don't take a holier-than-thou attitude about these alternative treatments," he emphasizes. "I realize we make our livings at this. But these clinics that operate offshore or in foreign countries are usually designed to make money.

"They do things to make people feel better, such as giving patients nicotine." As a matter of fact, in 1979 a surgeon reportedly passed himself off to Dr. Alivizatos as a patient and smuggled out a small sample of the mysterious serum. Analyzed in a University of Washington laboratory, it was found to contain pure nicotinic acid—nicotine.

"I don't think these clinics are altruistically attempting to cure people," Dr. Smithson continues, "they're perpetrating a scam. We [the medical establishment] may not have The Answer, but at least we go about our research in a legal, ethical way, with intellectual honesty."

While I do feel the U.S. Food and Drug Administration can be maddeningly slow to approve and make available promising new drugs, I simply do not subscribe to the notion that the National Cancer Institute and its counterparts are deliberately quashing alternative methods of cancer care. Does anyone truly believe that if some magical cure existed, physicians sworn to preserving human life would withhold it from their patients?

Organizations such as FACT and IACVF should be commended for spreading valuable information on cancer prevention and for advocating a patient's freedom of choice with regard to treatment options. But it seems to me their wholesale acceptance of modalities that have not undergone rigorous, well-controlled testing and review is motivated less by sound scientific reasoning than by the desperate cry of their constituents, many of whom face certain death. It is easy to understand why a terminal patient would respond eagerly to a healer promising life rather than to a physician who frankly concedes, "There's nothing else we can do."

Guidelines When Considering Alternative Therapies

Proponents of unconventional treatments frequently:

- Boast fanciful degrees (Doctor of Naturopathy, Doctor of Metaphysics) not recognized by legitimate institutions.
- Cry persecution by the established medical community and regulatory agencies.
- Claim their methods produce no adverse side effects. This alone obviously has tremendous appeal to cancer sufferers. The truth is, a patient's quality of life when following many holistic, "natural" approaches often compares unfavorably with that of patients treated by traditional medicine.

  A 1991 study published in the *New England Journal of Medicine* found that of 156 patients with advanced cancer, those treated conventionally at the Hospital of the University of Pennsylvania consistently reported a significantly more satisfying and pain-free existence than those given alternative therapy (consisting of a vegetarian diet, enemas, and a vaccine that purportedly boosts the immune system) at the Livingston-Wheeler Clinic in San Diego.
- Distort facts or offer scanty proof of their successes. For example, with the Greek Cancer Cure, diagnosis is made not through a definitive biopsy but through a less conclusive blood test. It is quite possible that some of Dr. Alivizatos's cancer patients were "cured" of a disease they never had. Too, inflated accounts of patients restored to health by

way of alternative means often neglect to mention that these people were simultaneously receiving standard treatment.

Proponents of unconventional treatments rarely:

• Have an affiliation with recognized teaching hospitals or universities.
• Disclose thorough records of their patients, their treatment methods, or the substances (vitamins, serums, and so forth) they use.
• Report their findings in one of the thousands of respected medical or scientific journals but rather in promotional materials designed to bedazzle the layman. These often contain glittering testimonials from satisfied clients, celebrities, and doctors—none of them trained in oncology.

We advise disregarding any treatment that promises it alone can cure your child and advocates abandoning approved therapy, or attempts to deposit responsibility for the cancer on the patient. Maintaining a positive attitude can certainly aid recovery, but I find those philosophies that invest patients with an unrealistic degree of control over their illnesses potentially destructive. How marvelous for the person who survives, but what about those who don't? Who must now go to their graves bearing the additional burden of guilt, feeling they somehow failed themselves.

This is too critical a decision to be made indiscriminately. Before you proceed with any alternative treatment, get the facts. In addition to obtaining the American Cancer Society's in-depth reports on unproven treatments, dig up studies and articles at your local library. A librarian can show you how to use the *Reader's Guide to Periodical Literature,* a standard reference book that indexes magazine pieces by subject; for instance, under "Cancer Therapy." Many medical libraries and university libraries carry *Index Medicus,* a reference index of thousands of medical and scientific journals such as the aforementioned *New England Journal of Medicine* and the *Journal of the American Medical Association.* These and others routinely report on unconventional cancer treatments.

Most important of all, discuss the prospective treatment method with your child's physician. Some parents worry that raising this issue will be taken as a criticism of the present standard treatment. No matter how outlandish—I don't care if you hand your doctor an article touting

"The Amazing Anchovy and Applebutter-Jelly Cancer Cure"—he should respond seriously to your questions.

"It's not fair to offhandedly pooh-pooh it," says Dr. Gilchrist, who listens to parents' inquiries all the time. "The physician has got to give the individual the opportunity to talk about it and to receive a reasonable critique."

Dr. Bringelsen concurs, explaining, "I usually try to anticipate questions about alternative treatments in our initial talks. I tell parents that they'll hear all kinds of things from a lot of well-meaning people, from 'How could you possibly give your child chemotherapy?' to offers of 'monkey juice,' or what have you. If they are interested in these therapies, they should bring me whatever they've read about it, so that we can take a look at it and discuss it together.

"If it's something that could supplement the treatment we're giving, and they feel strongly about it, I usually don't see any harm. For example, a vitamin that won't interfere with chemotherapy. Here in Virginia, where I practice now, we have a lot of mountain folk who want to use herb remedies, and that's okay.

"But if it's just absolute nonsense," she continues, "I'll tell the parents so. Sometimes they will ask about something that's so far out, they'd really be wasting their money more than anything. And I'd hate for them to do that. Or to travel around with a sick child who should not be going places."

A well-intentioned woman whose son died from cancer once sent me an article suggesting that cold pureed asparagus might provide a cancer cure. I immediately thrust it in front of one of Jason's resident doctors at the Mayo Clinic.

"Well, there is some medical foundation to what they're saying," he said, perusing the clipping. "Asparagus contains a particular property used in the drug asparaginase to treat leukemia. But the article is greatly oversimplified. Geralyn, do you realize how much asparagus you would have to give Jason for it to have any therapeutic value?

"We can't say that it's going to help him," he added doubtfully, "but it isn't going to harm him either."

That was all I needed to hear. Over the next couple of days I pureed canned asparagus and chased my son around the house with spoonfuls of the mud-green stuff. He swiftly ended my experimental study by refusing to swallow a single bite.

Where life-saving measures are concerned, I think any parent would go to extraordinary lengths. You'd crawl to hell and back if somebody told you that's what it took to get an edge. But when considering unproven treatments, observe this rule of thumb: if it sounds too good to be true, it probably is.

PREOPERATIVE PROCEDURES

The week leading up to his surgery, slated for the second Tuesday in September, Jason was sicker and weaker than ever. Two Fridays before, his schoolteacher phoned me in the middle of the afternoon. "Jason is so tired, he can hardly keep his head up," she said worriedly. I immediately drove down there and brought him home.

Over the next eight days he suffered intermittent fever and extreme fatigue, the result of alarmingly low blood counts from his previous chemotherapy treatment and the lingering aftereffects of radiation. At one stretch Jason slept twenty out of twenty-four hours, barely able to rouse himself to consciousness.

He did manage to stay awake long enough to sit through critical daily blood tests. According to Jason's doctors, surgery could not be performed until his white counts returned to normal, due to the risk of infection. For that reason they decided to discontinue chemotherapy until after the operation. It was a nerve-racking time. While we waited for the white-blood-cell levels to rise, were malignant cells multiplying inside of him, having been granted this temporary reprieve?

The low point came the day before we were to leave for Rochester. I remember sitting slumped on the living-room floor beside the sofa where Jason slept. As I listened to his faint breathing, I mournfully watched his narrow chest rise and fall, not sure if it would rise again.

My God, I thought to myself, *are we doing the right thing, putting Jason through so much suffering?* The doctors, while hopeful, could offer no guarantees concerning our son's survival. *What if he dies anyway? Look at what we've done to him.* That was the only time I ever second-guessed consenting to this grueling treatment.

What if Jason hadn't responded to therapy, like his friend Jill? The brave little girl's Burkitt's lymphoma returned once, twice, then a third time, infiltrating her central nervous system. "This isn't working, is it?" her mother bluntly asked one of the doctors.

"No, it's not," the physician admitted, "and we're running out of options."

When the next dose of chemotherapy proved ineffective at staving off the cancer, Jill's parents and the medical team mutually agreed that further therapy would only impair the quality of the little time that she had left. And to what end? The family took their six-year-old daughter home, so that she could at least spend her final days in familiar, comfortable surroundings.

At what point should treatment be discontinued? Only a child's parents can make that difficult decision, weighing such factors as the prognosis, the degree of the patient's suffering, and their personal beliefs concerning death and dying and quality of life. One set of parents might believe that life is sacred at any cost, while another might agree with Jason's remark "There's worse things than dying."

Though it's hard to predict your response in a given situation, I can't see my husband and me having withdrawn our son from treatment unless we'd exhausted every medical option. Even then, I just don't know. It's very, *very* difficult to imagine us ever having given up. Thank God we never had to render such a decision.

Sunday morning, on our way to Saint Marys Hospital, we dropped off Tim and Adam at our friends' farm just outside Worthington. Ron and Sarah had generously volunteered to take the two for the week. We hadn't been there thirty minutes when Tim ran inside the house, screaming and crying. While playing in a barn hayloft, he'd lost his footing and fallen through an opening, blackening his eyes and breaking his nose. *What else?* I thought.

By now Jason was such a veteran of medical facilities, he probably should have been awarded an honorary surgical mask and scrub suit at admission. Had this been his first trip to the hospital, we would have requested a brief orientation tour. At many centers a nurse or social worker will escort new patients and their families through the building, letting young people visit the operating and recovery rooms and fiddle around with stethoscopes and other medical instruments. They may also meet with the surgical team, who will answer questions and show the child what they will be wearing the next time she sees them.

In addition arrangements can be made for youngsters to talk to someone who has weathered the same type of surgery, while patients about to undergo an amputation can handle the prosthesis they will have to wear. Similarly kids scheduled to lose a leg can practice walking with crutches, which they will need for a time. Studies show that children prepared mentally prior to an operation are often less anxious afterward.

The pediatric surgeon, Dr. Bruce Kaufman, stopped into Jason's room. He was a surprisingly young man, about our age, with a full head of dark, curly hair. Conditioned to expect the TV stereotype from central casting—silver-haired, distinguished-looking, fatherly—Craig and I were somewhat startled the first time we met him. We exchanged glances as if to say, *He's the surgeon?*

Personable and reassuring, Dr. Kaufman patiently described to Jason what he could expect, tracing a line across our son's abdomen to show him where the incision would be made. Later my husband and I went over this and other points with Jason. Prior to surgery, both parents and their young patient should know the following details:

- How long the operation is expected to take. However, remember that if a surgery lasts longer than anticipated, it's not necessarily an indication that something's gone wrong. An earlier surgery might have run late, for example. Don't panic if it exceeds the physician's estimate.
- Where the child will wake up (the recovery ward? the intensive-care unit?) and whether or not his parents will be permitted to visit.
- The location and intensity of any anticipated discomfort or pain.
- The likelihood of reactions, such as nausea and vomiting, cramps, or weakness.
- The form of pain relief to be administered and its side effects.
- Whether he will require intravenous lines, catheters, feeding tubes, or transfusions.
- Approximately how long the patient will be hospitalized.
- Approximately how long he will be bedridden at home.
- The degree to which the surgery will disable or disfigure the patient, if at all.

In private Dr. Kaufman sketched the best- and worst-case scenarios. Hopefully, he said, the cancer was confined to the visible tumor. But there were several complications. For one, the lump definitely had invaded Jason's intestines, part of which would have to be removed. Because our son's diminished white counts left him susceptible to infection, in the seventy-two hours before surgery he was given about thirty enemas—no exaggeration—to clear the intestinal tract of germs and bacteria.

"Should the colon also be involved," the surgeon went on, "we will have to take it out immediately." Naturally the thought of our six-year-old wearing a colostomy bag for the rest of his life upset us. But it was certainly preferable to the gravest possibility, that microscopic malignant cells had disseminated to other vital organs and that Jason would soon die. There was no way to predict what he would find, Dr. Kaufman said.

Some parents still believe the superstitious old wives' tale that cutting open a patient with cancer is like stirring up a swarm of restless bees. According to Nurse Betcher, "I even used to hear that in nurse's training." Rest assured that it is pure fallacy.

Strange as it may sound, when Jason's physicians first informed us they planned to operate, I was elated, almost relieved. As long as his abdominal tumor still darkened the ultrasound monitor week after week, I could not persuade myself our son would survive. "I felt the same way," says Craig. After three months of intolerable uncertainty and tension, "The operation was going to tell us one way or the other."

The results of Jason's last blood test, taken Saturday in a Worthington lab, showed that his white count had climbed back into an acceptable range. But when tested the next day at Saint Marys, the level of *neutrophils*, a type of white blood cell, had dropped, postponing surgery and winding everyone's nerves that much tighter. Monday they drew another sample. Too low. Then again on Tuesday. This time there were enough neutrophils to proceed with the operation the next morning.

Anesthesia

One to several days before surgery you will meet with the *anesthesiologist,* a physician whose duties include prescribing the drugs and the method of anesthesia. During surgery he either administers anesthesia personally or supervises a nurse called an *anesthetist,* trained in this procedure.

After examining your child, the anesthesiologist will ask you about her medical history, allergies, all current medications, and any previous operations. I mentioned that when Jason had his oral surgery in June, the gas used to put him under made him quite ill afterward. The doctor took down this information, which would influence the type of anesthesia he and the surgeon selected:

• *General*—the most potentially dangerous method, it hastens the patient into unconsciousness. General anesthesia may be injected directly into the bloodstream or, in gas form, it may be inhaled.

• *Regional*—anesthetic agents are injected into part or parts of the body, interfering with the ability of nerves in that area to transmit pain impulses to the brain.

• *Local*—similar to regional, but affects a smaller area; primarily for minor surgery.

• *Spinal*—a needle delivers the drugs to the spinal-cord sac, blocking sensation in the pelvis and legs. *Epidural* anesthesia, often used in childbirth, is also injected into the back, but outside the spinal canal. While not as thorough, its postsurgery side effects are generally less uncomfortable.

• *Topical*—an anesthetic is sprayed or brushed on the area. Sometimes used in conjunction with local anesthesia, this technique is often employed for procedures involving the eyes, nose, or throat.

Although anesthesia is safer than ever, it is not without risk. It's impossible to foretell every patient's response, and the operating team must be ready to handle an emergency at a second's notice. A simple oversight or miscalculation in the operating room can seriously harm, even kill, a patient. Anesthesia is really an art of balance. The anesthesiologist must ensure that the patient remains sedated through the procedure yet receives enough oxygen to prevent brain damage or death.

Insist that the person recording information about your youngster be an anesthesiologist, not an anesthetist, a nurse, or other health-care worker. Be sure that this anesthesiologist will be attending your child in surgery. If not, demand to meet with whoever will be. Then ask:

- What type of anesthetic will you be giving my child?
- What are its side effects and risks?
- What type of medication will my child receive before he's taken into surgery?
- Will you be administering the medication and anesthesia or will an anesthetist?
- How long after surgery will my child regain consciousness?

Preparation Before Surgery

Throughout the rest of Tuesday Jason was prepped for surgery. Every few hours a lab technician came around to take blood and urine samples and to check his blood pressure. To prevent infection, an intravenous line delivering antibiotics was inserted into his hand.

So that patients will not vomit and choke while under anesthesia, they must fast twelve hours or more before the operation. A note will be posted on your child's bed, and, if he is ambulatory, on his pajamas, reading "NPO"—an abbreviation for the Latin expression meaning "Nothing by Mouth."

Because Jason was undergoing abdominal surgery, it was critical that his intestines be empty. Therefore he couldn't eat or drink any food or liquid once he entered the hospital. Instead he received various nutrients and fluids through the I.V. If Jason hadn't been so exhausted, this might have presented a problem. Fortunately he slept much of the time. For a youngster who complains of hunger, there is little you can do other than to shut the door to his room around mealtime, so that he doesn't smell or see the trays of food for the other patients.

The following procedures, too, may be carried out before the operation:

- Shaving around the area, if necessary.
- X rays.
- *Electrocardiography* (ECG or EKG). In this test, similar to electroencephalography (EEG), electrodes are attached to the body. A machine

called an electrocardiograph traces on paper the rhythm and other actions of the heart.

- Insertion of a catheter into the bladder, for patients who may not be able to urinate on their own following surgery.
- Insertion of a stomach tube, through either the mouth or the nostrils, for infusing liquid food or for quelling nausea and vomiting.

The period prior to surgery is another one of those times when parents should be at their child's side. That night I slept next to Jason's bed once again, while Craig took up his usual residence in the activity room.

Wednesday morning, says Jason, "I tried to stay asleep as long as I could. I didn't want to wake up, because I was afraid something might happen in the middle of the operation." According to the National Cancer Institute, kids typically worry about the anesthesia, pain, disfigurement, and if their parents will be at their bedside when they regain consciousness.

I'd always assumed that, like adults, youngsters would fear never waking up from the anesthesia. But based on the countless phone calls Jason has received from young cancer patients, the opposite appears to be true. I can't tell you how many kids facing surgery have anxiously asked Jason if he'd known anyone who woke up in the middle of the operation to find the surgeon cutting away. Jason always assures them they don't have to worry about that grisly scenario.

All in all, our son was actually quite calm. A nurse at Saint Marys remarked that she'd never seen a more relaxed child. When they came to place Jason on the gurney and wheel him down to surgery, he was still snoozing.

I wish *I'd* been half as composed. Once Jason disappeared behind a pair of swinging doors, Craig and I began our vigil in a windowless waiting room on the surgical floor. How plain and austere it was: stark-white walls, green plastic chairs, no paintings, no magazines. Nothing to distract you from your anguish.

A small group of our relatives waited upstairs on the sixth floor. The only other people with us in the room were my teenage nephew, Jesse, and my older brother, Mike, in from California. "Sonny," we call him, because of his unfailingly upbeat disposition. Every so often he broke the heavy silence with words of encouragement.

Craig didn't need any pep talks. "I felt pretty confident that everything was going to be all right," he recalls. "I remember telling Geralyn that, and she looked at me and asked, 'How can you be so positive?' I don't know, but I honestly believed the doctor was going to come back with good news."

Not me, which, again, was indicative of our disparate attitudes throughout. I don't think of myself as a pessimist, but I was absolutely terrified that the surgeon was going to open Jason up and discover cancerous growths that had eluded his doctors.

"We really didn't know what we were going to find," says Dr. Gilchrist. "Generally we have the surgeon go back in only if we think that whatever is there is operable. Still, we remain uncertain until the surgeon actually inspects the situation.

"That is the moment of truth, and as you can imagine, it is very stressful. In Jason's case we had no way of knowing whether or not there were still cancer cells in the enlarged lymph nodes until after they had been removed and examined under the microscope."

I'd brought a Danielle Steel paperback with me, but would absent-mindedly leaf through several pages, then realize I hadn't digested a single word. Craig, meanwhile, nearly wore a furrow in the floor from pacing back and forth. Mostly the four of us just sat there absorbed in our own thoughts, anxiously waiting.

CHAPTER THIRTEEN

COUNTDOWN TO RECOVERY

Postoperative Care • Camps for Young Cancer Patients
• Side Effects from Discontinuing Chemotherapy

The door to the waiting area burst open, and Dr. Kaufman, still in surgical garb, hustled into the room. "The surgery is all over," he said, taking a chair. "Jason is in recovery and doing just fine."

And . . . ? Craig, Mike, Jesse, and I gaped at him, holding our breaths. I remember searching his inscrutable face for a clue.

"Well," he said, removing his glasses and rubbing his eyes, "there was one other possibility I didn't discuss with you. And the reason I didn't was because I didn't want to get your hopes up. There was a possibility—a slight possibility—that we could have found what we call a 'dead' tumor, meaning that the mass is still present but there are no live cancer cells within.

"And that is exactly what we found!"

"What does that mean?" my husband asked cautiously.

"That the medicine is very effective for Jason," the surgeon said, breaking into a smile. "I saw no live cells anywhere." In other words our son was in remission, with no detectable sign of cancer.

Recalls Craig, "It was like getting the wind knocked out of you." The four of us bounced out of our chairs, ecstatically embracing and kissing one another. My husband had a jubilant grin on his face, not to mention a new best friend in Dr. Kaufman.

With tears in my eyes I blurted, "Doctor, did you ever have a mother kiss you?"

"No." Pause. "But I wouldn't mind starting now!"

As the surgeon got up to leave, my brother, Mike, stuck out his hand. "Doc," he said, "I really want to thank you for not being a plumber."

POSTOPERATIVE CARE

After relaying the good news over the phone to Craig's mother, the boys, and several others, we joined our relatives for a celebratory lunch. Everyone had been too jittery that morning to eat much of a breakfast, so we gave the waitress quite a workout.

Craig and I then returned to Saint Marys, anxious to see Jason. "You can visit him in about four hours," we'd been told, "once he's been transferred from recovery to pediatric intensive care." With evening about to fall, the hospital corridors were quiet. By contrast, the ICU pulsed with activity and blazing lights. Craig and I squinted from the glare as a nurse led us to the room Jason shared with another little boy.

"I'm afraid you can't stay any longer than ten minutes or so," she instructed us.

Anesthesia usually wears off one to three hours following surgery. Jason's eyes were open, and he stirred uncomfortably, nauseous from the anesthesia and obviously in some pain. "We held off sedating him so that you could see him while he was still awake," the nurse explained.

"It's all over, honey," I whispered. "And we have wonderful news. The doctor said he couldn't see any cancer anywhere, and you're going to get better." Jason appeared to understand, but two days later would not remember having heard what I'd said. Soon the nurse was tapping my shoulder and saying we'd have to step outside, as they were about to sedate Jason. That night I bedded down on a sofa in the ICU waiting area, while Craig retired to—where else?—the sixth-floor activity room.

Thursday evening, orderlies wheeled Jason back to his room. The doctors had prepared us for what to expect, but the sight of a child's body tethered to his bed by tubes is always upsetting. In addition to a gastric-decompression tube that ran up our son's nose and into his stomach, Jason wore one catheter to drain the eight-inch-long incision and one for urine. As an unanticipated consequence of surgery, his bladder wasn't functioning properly—a temporary condition, his doctors reassured us.

Aside from the expected soreness in his midsection, Jason suffered few typical postsurgery side effects: gas pains, weakness, dizziness, and/ or headaches. By Friday he was feeling well enough to sit up and examine his scar, which he proudly showed off to anyone who was interested. And to those who weren't, come to think of it.

My son was so absorbed in tracing the stitches that ran practically from hip to hip, he barely reacted when I repeated the physicians' encouraging words. Over the last two days Drs. Gilchrist, Smithson, and Burgert had each dropped by to check on Jason and discuss his condition. All three sounded extremely pleased and considerably more confident about his chances for recovery.

This information merited only Jason's nonchalant "Oh, good!" He now admits to being more excited than he let on. "It was a big relief to know that I wouldn't have to fight as hard," he recalls. "And from then on, when I had spinals and stuff that hurt, I could think to myself, *This spinal is helping me get closer and closer to my goal.*"

I remember Dr. Burgert's visit in particular. Usually rather serious and proper, he grinned broadly as he strode into the room. "Got a beautiful, sunshiny morning today, don't we?" he exclaimed.

Oh, yes we do! Everyone's hearts felt light.

Except Adam's and, especially, Tim's. They missed their brother terribly. Craig had returned to Worthington once Jason was back in his room, and the following weekend he brought the boys with him to Rochester. By then neither had seen Jason in two weeks. But due to Jason's deficiency of white blood cells, a condition called *leukopenia,* the nurse on duty forbade them to visit him. I implored her to at least let the two peek into Jason's room, just to know their brother was all right. "No," she snapped, "rules are rules."

Another nurse resourcefully came up with a solution. "How about if I put a surgical mask over Jason's face, wrap him in a blanket, and wheel him up to the roof? That way your other sons can see him, and with the fresh air blowing there'll be little chance of exposing him to germs." Which is exactly what we did. The three boys were briefly reunited on the sunny, windy terrace of Saint Marys Hospital, laughing together and playing with their G.I. Joes.

After two weeks of hospitalization Jason was shuffling up the walk to our front door, still hunched over, but smiling and waving to his dad, brothers, and little sister. Within two days he was back at school, which seemed to have an invigorating effect. Already he looked better, the color having returned to his face, and I could see him growing noticeably stronger each day.

Today, says Dr. Gilchrist, "We might have declared Jason out of the woods following surgery. We now know with this type of tumor that if everything is still under control at the end of six months, you've probably won the battle." In 1984, despite intensive chemotherapy and radiation and two surgeries, our son faced another eighteen months of maintenance drug treatment (the same drugs, minus daunomycin, in reduced dosages) to intercept stray cancer cells.

Though optimistic, Craig and I realized our family's crisis was far from over. Jason continued to suffer the intolerable side effects of chemotherapy, including a new one: debilitating joint cramps. Submerging him in a hot—and I mean *hot*—tub of water was the only remedy for easing the pain.

Once, when it was my turn to be hospitalized at Saint Marys for a chronic back problem, Craig's mother stayed with the children. Jason had one of his spasms that night.

"I thought Jason was about to die," Grandma Gaes remembers. "He was throwing up, his bones all ached so. You couldn't touch him anywhere. I rocked him, I held him. I didn't know what to do. It was scary. By the time Craig came home, I was crying, Jason was crying. I couldn't take it."

June 28, 1985, marked a year since Jason's diagnosis. It was not yet the sort of anniversary that called for a celebration, but there were plenty of smiles around our home that day. For Jason's doctors had told us that if he survived one year without a relapse, his chances for recovery doubled.

Our son no longer resembled the sick little boy of six months earlier, his hair having regrown to its former length, and then some. Patients often find it comes back thicker than before, or a slightly different shade or texture. We noticed no such changes with Jason, whose blond, stick-straight locks began appearing as stubble around Christmastime.

"It came in bit by bit and looked *real* bad," he recalls, "one hair here, one hair there. Once it finally all came in, I decided not to cut it." Indeed, by summer it was on the shaggy side, hanging down his neck in a tail. In the past I might have ordered my son to the barber. Now, as far as I was concerned, he could look like Rapunzel if he wanted. It was just so wonderful to have the "old" Jason back. All these visible positive changes, I admit, made it easier for me to treat him like a normal, healthy child.

CAMPS FOR YOUNG CANCER PATIENTS

Even so, I trembled at the thought of sending Jason to a week-long sleepaway camp for young cancer patients that August. Indicative of the strides made in pediatric-cancer treatment, these camps are a relatively recent phenomenon, springing up in numbers only since the early 1980s. Before then simply not enough children survived the disease to create much of a demand.

There are approximately one hundred such camps throughout the country, in over forty states. The one Jason attended, Camp Courage, in Maple Lake, Minnesota, is for patients and their siblings. Other camps sponsor all-day and sleepaway programs for patients only, for siblings only, and for families. Many of those in warm climates offer sessions virtually year-round.

With few exceptions the camps have medical personnel on duty twenty-four hours a day and facilities for administering chemotherapy. Camp Courage, for instance, was staffed by several Mayo Clinic physicians, as well as other health-care professionals. Nevertheless at first I strenuously opposed Jason's attending the camp, a five-hour drive from Worthington. What if he hurt himself? Or suffered a delayed reaction to his previous chemotherapy treatment? I rattled off a whole laundry list of what-ifs.

"We sure got into a heated discussion on that one," Craig reflects with a chuckle. Once again, the two of us faced off on the issue of setting limits, with Craig taking the more lenient position. Ultimately Jason himself persuaded me to set aside my reservations and let him enroll.

It turned out to be such a fabulous experience that he returned the next three summers.

Jason describes camp as "a real fun place where you got to do pretty much what you wanted. There was swimming, hiking, camping, canoeing, sports, drama, photography, horseback riding. The camp even had its own greenhouse and zoo. I still stay in touch with some of the kids I met there."

Nestled in the woods, Camp Courage looks like a typical sleepaway camp, except that some of the seventy or so campers are bald or on crutches or mentally impaired. Or perfectly healthy. Perhaps the most enduring benefit, besides the activities and the fun, was getting to know other children of different ages and at various stages of recovery. Jason's cabinmates included kids from six to seventeen, some of whom were obviously ill, and others who were fully cured.

"That was real encouraging," says Jason, "to see that not everybody who gets cancer dies. And you learn a lot from one another, which helps you to deal better with your own situation." The last summer he went, 1988, our son had been finished with treatment for over two years and was able to counsel other boys.

On the other hand, seeing kids in wheelchairs, for instance, never seemed to have a depressing effect on him. Jason understood from his own experience that another camper's sickly appearance was not necessarily indicative of his condition.

Being away from home gives young patients a chance to develop independence, a precious commodity for kids who've been so dependent for so long. The experience also proved valuable for my husband and, especially, me, showing us that we could relinquish our child to someone else's care without falling apart. We sent postcards back and forth that week ("The pizza's good, but they make us eat vegetables," grumbled one of Jason's), but I resisted the temptation to call him.

When we picked him up on Sunday, he was excited to see us and proud that he'd lasted the week. Frankly I wasn't sure that he would. "He was lonesome at first," the head counselor told us, "but he got into the swing of things and did real well." Counselors at these camps are usually eighteen and older, and many are health-care professionals. Jason's counselor, a college student named Troy, remains one of his best friends.

Most cancer camps are free to state residents, with a minority charging a nominal tuition of around fifty dollars. For a free national directory of children's cancer camps, published by Ronald McDonald Children's Charities, write or call Children's Oncology Camps of America, Inc., care of Dr. Edward S. Baum, M.D., Box 30, The Children's Memorial Hospital, 2300 Children's Plaza, Chicago, Illinois 60614, (312) 880-4564.

WHEN A CHILD
DIES OF CANCER

That October our son, who was still steadily improving, celebrated his eighth birthday. When a child has cancer, a tinge of dread can color even the happiest of times. With two thirds of all young cancer patients dying from the disease, Jason's medical progress often made me pause to reflect on what might have been.

Some nights, especially early in treatment, I would imagine him dying. During the day you are so preoccupied with caring for your youngster, you have neither the time nor the mental energy to contemplate the myriad of possibilities. Now and then, with the kids asleep and the lights out, I'd lie in bed and envision a future without Jason. What would normally joyful occasions, such as Timmy's confirmation, Adam's wedding, or Missy's elementary-school graduation, be like? I'd picture myself stammering to a stranger that Craig and I had *three* children instead of four. . . .

Perhaps subconsciously I was trying to prepare myself for the worst. Parents who have lost a child to a lingering disease such as cancer often find that even though they have anticipated their youngster's dying for weeks, months, sometimes even years, death still comes as a shock.

"You're never prepared," says Susan Arleo, whose twenty-two-year-old son John succumbed to brain cancer after a four-year struggle. "I went through the entire ordeal with him—two surgeries, radiation, chemotherapy, endless CAT scans and blood tests, seizures—yet I never truly believed that he would die."

John Arleo's passing submerged Susan and her husband in grief, a prolonged and unpredictable process that affects mourners emotionally, physically, and socially. Grief is typically described as having three general components. First, denial and disbelief; followed by a stage of acute mourning, once the concerned relatives, friends, and neighbors have returned to their own lives and the reality of the death starts taking hold; then a gradual acceptance and resumption of normal everyday life.

"There is no one fashion of bereavement," emphasizes Mayo Clinic social worker Ginny Rissmiller, who is specially trained in grief counseling. "Parents may not go directly from phase one to phase two to phase three. Or they may vacillate among them.

"Grief is uniquely personal, and everybody grieves differently."

This includes mothers and fathers. In her experience at the Mayo Clinic, Ginny has found that in most instances "both parents will not mourn the same way." Generally "The men are reluctant to shed tears and tend to keep their emotions to themselves, believing this is what society expects them to do. Whereas the women lay out their emotions and cry."

Essential differences between two parents might have first manifested during the child's illness and then exacerbated as her condition worsened, creating a conflict serious enough to splinter a marriage. For example, the more outwardly emotional partner may accuse her less verbal spouse of indifference, when in reality his anguish is just as intense. Grief, we must stress, cannot be measured in spilled tears. Furthermore no one has the right to expect another mourner to conform to his or her ideas of "proper" grieving.

Couples must accept each other's ways of expressing and handling bereavement, regardless of how diverse. Susan Arleo observes that she and her husband, John, are "extremely different. He's a churchgoer and visits the cemetery all the time. I do neither. But we let each other do our own thing, and it's worked out very well."

Some studies have put the divorce rate among bereaved parents at more than four in five. To place that figure in perspective, many of those marriages probably suffered preexisting problems. The unions' already shaky foundations then crumbled from the stresses of children's cancer. How sad for one tragedy to be compounded by the further tearing apart of a family. Keep in mind that a youngster's passing need not spell the end of a basically solid marriage. With open communication and mutual sensitivity, grieving husbands and wives can cope with and endure this terrible time.

Common Reactions to a Loss

Grief entwines itself around every aspect of your life, from your rapport with others, to your concentration at work, to your self-image. It encompasses a broad range of emotions. Mourners may experience some or all of those presented here; again it should be stressed that every person's reaction to a loved one's death is uniquely personal.

Anger is an extremely common emotion among the bereaved. This is particularly true when the victim is a child, for a young person's passing can uproot our most deeply held assumptions about life. It is unnatural for a child to predecease her parents, and the inability to make sense of this injustice often arouses furious disillusionment.

Anger can show itself either through raging outbursts or, less violently, through pent-up bitterness and irritability. Mothers and fathers frequently seek someone or something to blame for their child's death and vent their frustration at the medical staff, God, even parents whose families are, in Susan Arleo's words, "intact."

"For a time," she admits, "I tried avoiding even my dearest friends whenever they talked about their children. It was just too painful, because our kids grew up together. I used to listen to them describe their children's progress, but I wasn't *really* listening, and afterward it made me feel bad about having those feelings."

Usually a mourner's anger is more abstract, directed at intangible targets such as the cancer itself, rather than at a specific person or thing. Yet some parents can't help feeling angry at the child, for having abandoned them. This in turn can stir up feelings of extreme guilt, another emotion typical of grieving mothers and fathers.

A surprising number of parents believe they genetically bequeathed the disease to their offspring. According to Ginny Rissmiller, "The parents feel so responsible for their child that after he or she dies, they often feel they must have done something 'wrong.' " These parents will rewind and play back their youngster's life, over and over, and wonder, *Did I do something wrong during my pregnancy? Was there anything we did while she was alive that we should have changed?*

"Of course," Ginny adds, "more than likely nothing that they or the child did caused his cancer."

Parents may also blame themselves for somehow having failed their son or daughter, or second-guess themselves for having consented to or refused certain medical procedures. In almost all cases these parents are guilty only of torturing themselves needlessly.

Other reasons for guilt in the wake of a child's death include emotions society says are unwarranted or "selfish," but in fact are normal:

• ***Feeling a Sense of Relief After His Dying***—A normal reaction in instances where the patient was suffering.

• ***Guilt over Grieving Silently***—Our expectations of how we will respond to a loved one's passing usually come more from books, movies, and television than from personal experience. A stoic parent may worry that others will disapprove of his manner and that his lack of tears, for example, somehow indicates a lack of love for his dead child.

• ***Feelings of Resentment***—Over the enormous reserves of emotion, finances, and time the disease consumed, all for naught.

• ***Guilt over Having Perhaps Pulled Away from the Child During His Illness***—To this day I wonder about the father of that twenty-one-year-old patient we met at the Northland House. Unable to face the reality that his daughter was dying, he immersed himself in work so that he "didn't have time" to visit her in the hospital. How must he feel now that she is gone?

Mourners also contend with what are termed secondary losses: for instance, the erosion of one's self-identity that may result from a child's death. We often view our kids as extensions of ourselves, living symbols of our societal value and worth. If they should die, a parent's own sense of self may be thrown into chaos.

Perhaps the clearest illustration of this would be a mother and father who lose their only child. Part of their very identity is destroyed. Is it appropriate for them to still refer to themselves as parents? For almost all bereaved single-child parents, the universal desire to leave some surviving mark on the world has been dashed. Who will carry on the family name? Will they ever get to be grandparents? Who will mourn them when *they* die?

"I tend to see two reactions with one-child parents," notes Ginny Rissmiller. "One is that they decide to never have any more children." These parents may assume the cancer was hereditary. Or perhaps they simply cannot face the pain of enduring a youngster's death ever again, no matter how remote. "The other response is to want to have another child right away," to reclaim their roles as mother and father.

One youngster's death also irrevocably alters the structure of his family. To analogize the family to the human body, it's as if a vital limb has been amputated. The survivors must carry on, but will never fully compensate for the missing part. Intrafamily relationships often change due to this misfortune, either strengthening or weakening.

"I've seen parents completely ignore their other children," says Ginny Rissmiller. "They've focused so much attention on the dying child for so long that at the end they feel emotionally and physically wiped out and have no energy left. It takes a long time to recharge. Unfortunately their communication with the other kids may break down." When that happens, neglected siblings may grow resentful, feeling that their parents don't care for them as much as they did their deceased brother or sister. As with divorce, it is a sad state of affairs when a family drifts apart following one member's death.

Another not unusual reaction is for parents to unreasonably expect their surviving kids to "replace" the deceased child. This can inflict severe psychological damage, blurring their identities and crippling their self-esteem. Mothers and fathers may also come to idealize the deceased brother or sister, further stirring resentment among the surviving siblings.

When a child dies, his parents mourn him not only in the present but the future as well. They grieve for the hopes and dreams they once had, which are now buried along with him. "That's the most painful part," says Susan Arleo, "the would-bes." She remembers her son with pride as highly popular and outgoing, a good student and a talented athlete.

"The shame of it all is that John really enjoyed life. My husband and I assumed he would be successful, and we wanted to be along for the ride." Losing John, she says sadly, was like losing part of her own future.

Since his death in 1988, "Nothing seems real. It's like this is not my real life anymore." Parents frequently complain of feeling confused, disorganized, and/or disoriented following a child's death. They drift about in a fog, getting lost in familiar places or not functioning at their usual level in the workplace.

All of these reactions, unless severe or prolonged, are normal. Parenting, after all, demands tremendous amounts of time, responsibility, and sacrifice. Suddenly the family routine is disrupted, and grieving mothers and fathers now have a void in their lives that only time and support from others can help them fill.

Physical Symptoms of Grief

Grief affects people physically as well as emotionally. It's been shown that states of profound sadness or despair can lower the body's resistance to disease, setting off ailments such as frequent colds. Therefore it is especially important for grieving parents to take care of themselves. Other potential physical effects include:

- Fatigue, lethargy, exhaustion
- Sleeplessness, restlessness
- Eating disorders; extreme weight loss or weight gain
- Chronic crying jags
- Difficulty breathing
- Chest pain
- Trembling, shaking, or palpitations
- Dizziness
- Greatly reduced or heightened sexual feelings

No Timetable for Mourning

Bereavement experts generally agree that a parent's grief over a lost child is the most intense and ongoing of all. The extent and length of time a mother or father, respectively, will mourn depend on such factors as:

- Their personal perception of the depth of the loss. For example, even though two parents may lose the same child, each has lost a different relationship and role.
- Their concepts about death, such as belief in an afterlife, and so on.
- The manner in which the loved one died (illness, accident, homicide, suicide).
- Their relationship with the deceased. One of the saddest circumstances is when a child—or anyone, for that matter—dies with crucial issues and conflicts left unresolved. Few human relationships are devoid of problems or friction, including that between a parent and a child. This especially applies to teenage patients. Naturally rebellious, they may have waged battle not only against their cancer but in search of their independence, frequently locking horns with Mom and Dad in the process.

- Their attitudes throughout the patient's illness. Were they open, honest, and realistic? Or were they incommunicative and in denial?
- Their own physical and emotional health.
- Support from friends, relatives, neighbors.

Just as there is no right or wrong way to mourn, no timetable exists. It may take two months or two years to recover. In Ginny Rissmiller's opinion, "I would say that grieving is usually measured in years rather than in months."

Nearly all parents, she says, find that "the first year is the hardest." Holidays and anniversaries—of the child's death, her birthday, the first day of school—may trigger an avalanche of depression. Some people find keeping up family traditions a comfort, whereas for others it dredges up painful memories. Obviously families must do whatever is most comfortable for all their members.

Don't expect your bereavement to ebb steadily and gradually. For no apparent reason you may experience a sudden surge of anguish. It could be stimulated by a particular song on the radio, an old photograph, or a favorite family vacation spot. Likewise, even after grief has relaxed its hold, it can unexpectedly swell again like a tidal wave, engulfing you.

According to Susan Arleo, "Anything can act as a reminder." For her the mere sight of a young man wearing a baseball cap turned backward reawakens memories of her late son. Three years after John's passing she evaluates her mourning this way: "You don't cry as much, but the feelings are always the same. You still expect them to come walking in the door."

While grief's duration varies from parent to parent, friends and relatives may have their own ideas about what constitutes "appropriate" limits on mourning. Others often allot bereaved parents an unrealistic period in which to recover, then grow impatient should the mother or father continue grieving. They may remark insensitively, "It's time to move on with your life," or "You should be over it by now," causing the already distressed parent to feel guilty as well.

Is there a point where sustained or profound mourning turns unhealthy?

Counseling and Support Groups

Grief showers those in mourning with pain, loneliness, anxiety, helplessness, sorrow, emptiness, frustration, despair. Parents who have lost a child may at times feel overwhelmed or worry that they are going crazy, when in fact their reactions to this torrent of unfamiliar and complex emotions are entirely normal.

But some degree of counseling and/or therapy is advisable for all family members. Ginny Rissmiller will generally counsel bereaved families, referring them to a specially trained Mayo Clinic psychologist if appropriate. Today most medical centers retain some kind of therapist on staff.

Some examples of situations that would warrant therapy include:

- Marital discord, which can arise from the issues raised earlier in this chapter, as well as from stress over family finances, sexual incompatibility, breakdown in communications, and so on
- Deteriorating intrafamily relationships
- A persistent obsession with the deceased child: for instance, turning her bedroom into a shrine; or an unhealthy need to cling to the past
- A general lack of control or inability to forge ahead
- Self-destructive behavior, such as alcohol or substance abuse, or suicidal feelings, which should *always* be taken seriously

Parents who've suffered the death of a child cry out for support and friendship. Unfortunately they may have been so consumed with grief that they now find themselves isolated from others. Or the reverse may be true, where well-intentioned family and friends simply do not know how to console the bereaved.

A youngster's passing frequently makes other adults uncomfortable, reminding them all too vividly that this tragedy can befall anyone. It is telling about our society's reluctance to address the issue of children and dying that we have the words *widow* and *widower* to identify grieving spouses but none for the parents of a deceased child. Ultimately one of the greatest sources of comfort are support groups, composed of parents who have experienced a common tragedy.

Had Jason not survived Burkitt's lymphoma, Craig and I probably would have sought out the Spencer, Iowa, chapter of the Compassionate Friends, a nonreligious self-help organization for bereaved parents and siblings. Its approximately 640 chapters nationwide vary greatly in size, but all provide measures of hope, strength, information, empathy, and friendship. No dues are required.

For the Arleos, attending monthly meetings has better enabled them to resolve their grief. "Just meeting people who understand helps," says Susan. "Because most people you meet socially, if they ask you how many children you have, aren't prepared to hear, 'I have one son, and another who died of cancer.' "

At the Compassionate Friends "We have a whole group of people who under ordinary circumstances never would have touched one another's lives. You all share the same pain. Everything you say, they nod their heads. So it's just a safe place to be." All members are encouraged to speak, but always voluntarily.

"It's a high price to have to pay for friendship," Susan adds, "but we've made some very lovely friends." The Compassionate Friends originated in England in 1969; its first U.S. group was founded in Miami three years later. To locate the branch nearest you, contact the national office at P.O. Box 3696, Oak Brook, Illinois 60522, (708) 990-0010.

Another recommended organization is the Candlelighters Childhood Cancer Foundation (1312 Eighteenth Street, N.W., Suite 200, Washington, D.C. 20036, 800-366-2223; 202-659-5136 in Washington, D.C.), which sponsors over three hundred support groups across the country, for siblings and parents alike.

Brothers and Sisters Grieve Too

A parent's natural inclination is to shield his kids from anything unpleasant or traumatic. But most experts in the field of bereavement would probably concur with Ginny Rissmiller's contention that adults tend to underestimate youngsters' capacity to comprehend and cope with death.

How well siblings will handle a brother's or sister's passing hinges not only on their ages and level of maturity but on their involvement throughout the deceased's illness. "I have noticed," Ginny says, "that the kids who cope best are those who were included during treatment." Feeling helpless can be as agonizing for young people as for adults.

Michael Arleo was thirteen at the time of his older brother's cancer diagnosis. Over the next four years, says his mother, he assisted with John's home health care. "We approached this as a family, and Michael was a part of everything. He saw it all. John would eat at the dinner table, in his wheelchair, then Michael and I would bathe him and put him in bed." While this might not be practical with a younger child, helping his brother enabled Michael at least to exert some control and feel useful.

Should Siblings Attend the Funeral?

"Everybody asks that," says Ginny Rissmiller, adding that there is no set answer. "If you leave the other kids out," she cautions, "they're always going to wonder what was worth being so secretive about. Also, allowing them to take part in the funeral, even if in some small way, can help them to deal with their grief." However, children should never be forced to attend. One alternative for reluctant kids is to hold a private viewing or memorial for family members beforehand.

Adolescents, who usually want to be at their sibling's funeral, may wish to add their own personal touch, perhaps by sharing a poignant or humorous anecdote. Michael Arleo had one request of his parents: that his brother not be given a wake. "He didn't want everyone to remember John as sick," says his mother. Her husband, on the other hand, needed the ritual. In the end the family compromised. "We've got to do something for each of us," Susan told her son. "So instead of a three-day wake, we'll have just one day."

Depending on their ages, siblings will have to contend with any number of adult responses to bereavement, such as anger, guilt, and denial. Since they are inexperienced at surviving such tragedies, they will naturally be more fearful and confused. They may also act out in the ways we mentioned in Chapter Nine pertaining to a brother's or sister's serious illness: regressive behavior, bed-wetting, poor school attendance and/or performance, defiant behavior, "perfect" behavior.

One child's death may change the siblings' roles within the family—and consequently their self-identifies. For example, the second-oldest child may suddenly find herself the oldest and have to assume new responsibilities. Another may suddenly become an only child. Their mother and father may relate to them differently as well. In general a naturally turbulent time of life is made even more confusing.

To guide their children through this crisis, parents have to stay connected as best they can by encouraging them to discuss their feelings and fears, not only with Mom and Dad but with peers, grandparents, and other trusted friends. Yet parents must also recognize when their kids need private time for sorting out feelings.

In the aftermath of John Arleo's death, his mother admits, "I didn't know what was going in my son Michael's head; I didn't have time to ask him. And I still don't know if I'm ready to find out." When parents feel too overcome by grief to monitor their surviving children, I would suggest entering them in counseling or a sibling support group such as the Compassionate Friends or the Candlelighters. Their medical-center social worker can analyze the family's problems and make the appropriate referral.

Time, the Greatest Healer

"Time is such an important factor in working through grief," says Ginny Rissmiller. Yes, a child's death irrevocably changes a family, but eventually its members do usually manage to go on with their lives. While they desperately miss the deceased youngster, survivors often claim to sense his or her spiritual presence. Many parents draw solace from praying for their child, dreaming of them, talking to them, or communicating in some special, personal way.

"We have pictures of John all over the house," says Susan Arleo, "but I don't really need any reminders of him. He was a great one for putting his head on my shoulder, and I just feel it all the time. Wherever I go, I know he's with me, watching over me."

SIDE EFFECTS UPON DISCONTINUING MEDICATION

March 1986 brought another milestone—Jason's last chemotherapy treatment at the Mayo Clinic. A family album of photographs documents that final session: of Dr. Bringelsen smilingly examining him; Jason, clad in combat fatigues, hooked up to the I.V., about to receive his cyclophosphamide; Jason and Dr. Bringelsen ceremoniously shaking hands good-bye; then Jason striking a triumphant Rocky-like pose atop a stone wall outside the Mayo Building.

It was a day of mixed emotions. Though relieved for our son's sake, I was scared to let go of what had become our family's lifeline. I remarked anxiously to Dr. Bringelsen, "Jason's been getting along so well, do you think maybe we should continue the chemo for another six months? Just to be safe?"

She'd obviously heard this question before. "In all our studies," she replied patiently, "we've found that kids who are on chemotherapy for eighteen months survive just as long as kids who are on it for twenty-four. Doing this for another six months wouldn't cure Jason if he were not already cured. We think that this is the time to stop."

It may take up to a year for patients' bodies to adapt once chemotherapy drugs are discontinued. One night more than three months after his last dosage, Jason suddenly lost all feeling in both his legs, prompting another emergency trip to Saint Marys Hospital.

Almost eerily, again we had been at Grandma Gaes's in Storm Lake. Tired from a full day of swimming and playing, Jason lay down on the couch to watch the TV news, which happened to be broadcasting a feature on a pediatric-cancer survivor named Jason Gaes. When it was over, I turned off the set. "Okay, Mr. TV Star, time for bed."

Jason looked at me strangely. "I . . . I can't get up," he said. "My legs, they won't move."

My first thought was that a tumor in his spinal column was blocking the nerves. Just like two years earlier, Craig picked him up, rushed him out to the car, and drove to the office of our longtime family physician. After palpating Jason's spine for any obvious abnormality, Dr. Mailliard said, "I really can't tell you that it's not a tumor. I don't have the proper equipment here to diagnose it, so if I were you, I'd take him to Rochester and have them look at it there."

Fearing the worst, we retraced the familiar route, pulling up at Saint Marys Hospital around two o'clock in the morning. Craig and I were so exhausted that the staff gave us a gurney right next to Jason's there in the emergency room. I remember being awakened by the sound of several physicians examining Jason and whispering so as not to disturb us.

What they found wasn't a malignancy, thank goodness, but internal bleeding from where Jason had received his spinal injections. Dr. Smithson, consulting his notes, mused aloud that for three years in a row an emergency had arisen around this same time of year. Hugging me, he joked in a stern voice, "This is getting to be a habit, one that I would like you to break."

The following chart, adapted from the *USP DI, Volume II, Advice for the Patient* (copyright, the United States Pharmacopeial Convention, Inc., permission granted), lists the *potential* posttreatment side effects of agents commonly used to treat childhood cancer:

POTENTIAL SIDE EFFECTS UPON DISCONTINUING CHEMOTHERAPY THAT REQUIRE MEDICAL ATTENTION

Asparaginase	Severe stomach pain accompanied by nausea and vomiting
Bleomycin	Coughing; shortness of breath
Carmustine	Coughing; fever, chills, sore throat; shortness of breath; unusual bleeding or bruising
Chlorambucil	Coughing; fever, chills, sore throat; shortness of breath; unusual bleeding and bruising
Cisplatin	Impaired hearing; ringing in ears; fever, chills, sore throat; swollen feet or calves; unusual bleeding or bruising; unusually decreased urination
Cyclophosphamide	Bloody urine
Cytarabine	Fever, chills, sore throat; unusual bleeding or bruising
Dacarbazine	Fever, chills, sore throat; unusual bleeding or bruising

POTENTIAL SIDE EFFECTS UPON DISCONTINUING CHEMOTHERAPY THAT REQUIRE MEDICAL ATTENTION (cont.)

Dactinomycin	Black, tarry stools; diarrhea; fever, chills, sore throat; mouth or lip sores; stomach pain; unusual bleeding or bruising; jaundice
Daunorubicin	Irregular heartbeat; shortness of breath; swollen feet or calves
Dexamethasone	Abdominal, stomach, or back pain; dizziness, fainting; fever; continued appetite loss; nausea or vomiting; shortness of breath; unexplained headaches; unusual tiredness, weakness; unusual weight loss
Doxorubicin	Irregular heartbeat, shortness of breath; swollen feet or calves
Etoposide	None listed
Fluorouracil	Fever, chills, sore throat; unusual bleeding or bruising
Hydrocortisone	Abdominal, stomach, or back pain; dizziness, fainting; fever; continued appetite loss; nausea or vomiting; shortness of breath; unexplained headaches; unusual tiredness, weakness; unusual weight loss
Hydroxyurea	Fever, chills, sore throat; unusual bleeding or bruising
Lomustine	Fever, chills, sore throat; unusual bleeding or bruising
Mechlorethamine	Fever, chills, sore throat; unusual bleeding or bruising

POTENTIAL SIDE EFFECTS UPON
DISCONTINUING CHEMOTHERAPY THAT
REQUIRE MEDICAL ATTENTION (cont.)

Mercaptopurine	Fever, chills, sore throat; unusual bleeding or bruising; jaundice
Methotrexate	Blurred vision; convulsions or seizures; dizziness; headaches; confusion; fatigue, weakness
Plicamycin	Bloody or black, tarry stools; tiny red spots on skin; sore throat, fever; unexplained nosebleed; unusual bleeding or bruising; bloody vomit
Prednisone	Abdominal, stomach, or back pain; dizziness or fainting; fever; continued appetite loss; muscle or joint pain; nausea or vomiting; shortness of breath; fatigue, weakness; unusual weight loss
Procarbazine	Adverse reactions to foods high in tyramine content, such as cheese, soy sauce, and sour cream. (A more comprehensive list of these foods can be found in Chapter Five.)
Thioguanine	Fever, chills, sore throat; unusual bleeding or bruising
Vinblastine	None listed
Vincristine	None listed

When June 28 came around again, with Jason still in remission, we were ready to celebrate. On that day in 1986 we finally threw the party we'd imagined together so many times. The invitation—a photocopy of Jason's recently completed book about cancer, illustrated by his brothers—read:

"On June 28, 1984, our world was shattered when our six-year-old son, Jason, was diagnosed with a rare type of cancer and we were told there was a strong possibility that he would not be with us for his seventh birthday. With your loving support, the doctors' dedication and God's infinite mercy, Jason is now eight years old, strong in body and spirit, and is now at the end of his two years of treatment. Craig and I, the boys and Melissa ask you to come and celebrate with us. . . ."

Long before the hundreds of invitations went out that spring, the party had been a much-awaited event, not only for our family but for relatives and friends. "Everybody knew there would be this big party once Jason was done with treatment," remembers my mother, "and it became a constant topic of conversation. You'd talk to this one, and she'd say, 'I'm saving up for a new dress for Jason's party. I have it on layaway.' And then you'd talk to this one, and she'd tell you how she was going on a diet for the big day. It gave everyone something positive to look forward to."

A party where all the ladies wear new dresses and all the men drink beer. That had been Jason's wish, and we let him plan the affair as much as he wanted until it matched the one of his dreams. He had such fun selecting the menu, his dad's and brothers' outfits, even my dress. At the end of an unsuccessful shopping trip my mother and I were about to give up for the day when we shuffled wearily into J. C. Penney's.

Jason spotted a white satin sundress hanging on a sales rack. Examining it critically, he exclaimed, "I like this one!"

I flipped over the price tag. *Only six dollars?*

"Kid," I said, "you've got it."

For himself Jason chose a crisp white tuxedo, white ruffled shirt, and a fire-engine-red bow tie with matching cummerbund.

The party, held at the lakefront resort we belonged to in Okoboji, Iowa, surpassed all our expectations. Four hundred people packed the cavernous red-and-white festooned hall to eat, drink, and dance. Down the middle of the room ran five eight-foot buffet tables brimming with roast pork and beef and sixty-odd salads, all prepared by a committee of about a dozen women.

In attendance were friends, classmates of Jason's, relatives, and many of the medical personnel who'd participated in his recovery. "It was great," he remembers, "just everything a kid could want. The gigantic cake, the music." Anything else? "Oh, yeah, and the presents."

Twelve hours after it began, the disk jockey spun the final song of the evening, Frank Sinatra's "New York, New York." Everyone gathered in a circle, holding hands, and cheered as Craig hoisted our grinning son up in the air. Jason could have levitated on the love filling that room alone.

CHAPTER FOURTEEN

LIFE AFTER CANCER

Family Readjustment • Cancer Therapies of the
Future • Long-Term Side Effects of Treatment

As of March 17, 1987—the first anniversary of his last chemotherapy—
we've been able to say Jason *had* cancer rather than *has* cancer. According to his physicians, because he remained disease-free in that year, the
chance of our son dying of cancer is now only barely greater than that
of any child his age.

But is he cured? In most cases a patient is pronounced cured if still
in remission five years after either diagnosis or the end of treatment,
though with some cancers eight to ten years is considered a safer
margin. Despite the fact that our son has surpassed both five-year
marks, no doctor has ever said flat out, "Jason is cured."

Dr. Gilchrist explains why: "Jason is probably as cured as he's ever
going to be, so perhaps it's superstition on our parts that we don't say
'He's cured.' But we haven't been successful at this that long that we can
comfortably speak those words. We've been stung by the fact that with
some tumors everything was fine, and then suddenly the cancer re-
curred after five or more years."

ADJUSTMENTS IN FAMILY LIFE

Most pediatric-cancer survivors adjust well to life after their disease. For a time, however, it is not unusual for a kid to cling to his "patient" identity or to feel neglected now that Mom and Dad are paying attention to other family members and problems again. Jason freely admits that initially "I missed getting all the attention."

To reclaim it, kids may suddenly become dependent, or rebellious and defiant. This happened with our son. In the months after his final chemotherapy treatment Jason began misbehaving and talking back, which was so unlike him. If he flung his coat on a chair and I asked him to please hang it up, he'd snap, "Tim never hangs *his* up!" Concerned, I mentioned this to Nurse Betcher.

"A lot of kids go through that," she said. "Face it: he's been bombarded with attention for the past couple of years. Just give him lots of hugs and kisses, and it will work itself out." Which it did.

Parents, too, may face a difficult transition back to normal life. Strange as it might seem, some find themselves at loose ends without the all-consuming crisis that shaped and defined their lives. There is no question that such an ordeal can change you forever. As we discussed in Chapter Nine, the mother who becomes more independent in the course of overseeing her child's health care may resist returning to a traditional—and now confining—marriage where her husband makes all the decisions.

Some parents try to sustain their crisis-time roles by overprotecting their child, in effect rendering him the eternal patient. In a perverse way this ensures the child's continued dependence on Mom and Dad and prevents him from growing up. In Dr. Bringelsen's view the families that play out these scenarios are those that coped poorly throughout the youngster's illness.

"Some of the parents get so darned overinvolved with this that they can't let go and don't let the child develop into a healthy adult," she observes. "The families that are probably the healthiest are the ones who put it behind them and describe their child as having had cancer and don't dwell on him being a survivor."

Other common reactions parents may have to a child's recovery:

• Expecting perfection of the child, in an unconscious demand for a fair exchange for their months or years of sacrifice. This behavior is potentially harmful and requires the intervention of a hospital social worker or a family therapist should it persist.

• A profound sense of loss over the diminished contact with the physicians, nurses, and other medical-team members with whom they formed a special bond. These dedicated professionals care for parents as well as for their children. Although you still see them at routine checkups, the relationships will probably not be as intimate and will grow less so over time.

"It's hard to have a relationship with a family and then stop it," says Dr. Bringelsen, "but actually I think it's healthier for both of us that way. We follow the children for years after they recover, and that's real fun and special, to watch them grow. But there comes a time when you have to stop, usually around college age.

"It's frequently the parents who are tied to us more than the kids, who are tired of going to the doctor anyway! They don't realize the fear, anguish, and anxiety their parents went through early on, when the cancer was diagnosed."

Our family had little problem settling down to normal. However, things might have turned out differently had Jason's treatment been abruptly terminated rather than continued for eighteen months. During that year and a half the cancer remained a major focus, but not the only one. As his chances for survival steadily improved, we began doing more of the things we used to, such as participating in the other children's activities. By the time Jason finished, our family was more or less whole again.

After all this discussion about learning to put the crisis of pediatric cancer behind you, I must concede that Jason's disease is still very much a part of our life today. All because of a certain book originally scrawled in a yellow spiral notebook.

Ironically our son was aghast when I suggested we photocopy his book to serve as the invitation to his party. "Oh, no," he said. "No way."

"Why not?"

"Because grown-ups will laugh. I know I didn't spell some of the words right."

"I promise you, honey, nobody will laugh at your book. It's very good." He gave in, on the condition that Tim and Adam illustrate it, so that it looked more like a "real" book.

Several volunteers from the American Cancer Society were among Jason's many guests that day. They were so impressed with the book that the organization requested permission from Jason to distribute copies to young cancer patients because he'd so vividly captured the experience.

One thing led to another, and in 1987 a publisher issued *My Book for Kids with Cansur,* with a portion of the proceeds going to the American Cancer Society. Addressing young readers, Jason wrote, "If you get scared, you can call me. My number is . . ." The phone started ringing and hasn't stopped since. To date I'd say our son has received over a thousand calls from around the world. So far Jason's book has been translated into French, German, and Japanese.

"One time," he recalls, "this little boy called me all the way from Ireland, collect. I didn't mean to talk to him for too long, but before I knew it, we'd been on the phone an hour and a half. When I told my dad afterward, he just about fainted."

The book's publication initiated a chain of events that we never could have imagined. Requests poured in for Jason to appear on TV. At age ten he just didn't know you're supposed to be intimidated when a TV camera is trained on your face. With seconds to go before airtime, *Sonya Live in L.A.* host Sonya Friedman asked Jason, "Are you nervous?"

"About what?"

"Well," she said, smiling, "millions of people are going to be watching you. Doesn't that make you nervous?"

"Have you ever had a spinal?" Jason replied. "Now, *that*'ll make you nervous."

In a bizarre twist the disease that temporarily stole his childhood has indirectly granted Jason a lifetime's worth of memorable experiences. On behalf of the American Cancer Society, Ronald McDonald's Children's Charities, and other organizations, he has spoken around the country to children and adults alike.

No matter how many times I accompany him to large speaking engagements, I am continually amazed at his poise. He's addressed ten thousand cancer survivors in a Kansas arena; appeared before a U.S.

congressional luncheon concerning federal funding for cancer research; and sung a song specially composed for and about him, "Here I Am," on a European American Cancer Society telethon.

In 1988 he, singer Connie Haynes, and actress Jill Ireland were honored at the White House for their work on behalf of the American Cancer Society. During the Rose Garden ceremony, then President Ronald Reagan read excerpts from Jason's book. "I thought it was really neat," recalls Jason. Such were an eleven-year-old's priorities that receiving an American Courage Award from the President rates a mere "really neat," whereas meeting his beloved Dan Marino was "awesome!"

Yet Jason remains unaffected by it all, and every bit a kid. At an American Cancer Society dinner for one thousand guests, he was asked if he wanted to say a few closing words.

"Yes, I would." Jason rose from his seat on the stage, leaned into the microphone, and said, "Well, I'd like to say . . . if anybody doesn't want their cherry pie, I'll take it!"

That same year Jason and our family were the subjects of an Academy Award–winning documentary, *You Don't Have to Die*, broadcast on the Home Box Office cable channel. Amid all the celebrating the night of its December 5, 1988, premiere came a sobering reminder of what might have been. Jason's dear friend, Harlan, passed away from sarcoma after watching *You Don't Have to Die* on television. He was just twenty-two. Today Jason strives to be as much of an inspiration to other children as Harlan was to him.

FRONTIERS IN CANCER THERAPY

When Jason reaches twenty-two by the end of this century, an estimated one out of every thousand young adults will have been cured of cancer. Increasingly attention is being focused not only on the medical issues affecting cancer survivors but on social concerns such as job discrimination and affordable health and life insurance. If the cure rate continues to rise at its current pace, by the year 2000 four of every five pediatric-cancer patients will be saved.

Those youngsters will likely reap the benefits of several promising experimental therapies currently under investigation. (By "experimental," we mean treatments subjected to strict scientific testing and review, not the unproven alternative methods discussed in Chapter Twelve.)

Biological Therapy

Biological therapy, also known as immunotherapy, utilizes natural or synthetic substances to jump-start and strengthen the body's natural immune response. According to a National Cancer Institute report, these *biological response modifiers* may directly inhibit malignancies from growing or they may indirectly enable healthy body cells to control cancer cells. It is believed that, once perfected, comparatively small dosages of biologics will effectively treat cancer without producing severe toxic side effects.

Scientists have been researching biological therapy for some time. In 1957 two British scientists discovered *interferon,* a family of naturally secreted proteins that suppress or destroy tumor cells and stimulate the immune system. One obstacle is isolating and purifying biological response modifiers so that they can be utilized. But in clinical trials alpha interferon, derived from white blood cells and other sources, has shown significant antitumor activity, including a response rate in excess of 80 percent against certain lymphomas and leukemias.

Another type of immunotherapy uses *interleukins,* hormonelike substances produced by the body's lymphocytes. Interleukin 2 (IL-2), discovered at the National Cancer Institute in 1976, stimulates the growth and activity of various natural cancer-destroying blood cells. To date, IL-2 has been given to patients in over fifty clinical trials.

The medical team of Dr. Steven A. Rosenberg developed a method whereby patients were injected with IL-2, after which precursor cancer-killing cells were separated either from the bloodstream or from the surgically excised tumor. These cells were incubated in a laboratory and then injected back into the patient. Preliminary results with IL-2 have been encouraging, in particular against advanced kidney cancer and melanoma.

Dr. Rosenberg's newest experimental treatment, approved for clinical trials in 1990, involves *gene therapy.* Of the various cancer-killing cells, tumor-infiltrating lymphocytes (TIL) are especially effective because they produce a powerful compound that literally eats away at malignant cells. Therapy with TIL requires a comparatively low dosage and zeros in on the particular tumor from which it was taken. To multiply the production of this compound a hundredfold, physicians insert a pair of genes into the lymphocytes taken from the removed tumor and then transfer them back to the patient.

One other promising biologic, *monoclonal antibodies,* may act as an early-warning system and make possible early cancer diagnosis. These scientifically tailored proteins can locate and bind to cancer cells when the disease is most treatable, long before the onset of symptoms. Monoclonal antibodies are not known to kill tumorous cells by themselves. However, when combined with anticancer agents, they function as Trojan horses, delivering the cancer killers directly to the tumor.

Hyperthermia

Hyperthermia, which involves treating tumor cells with heat, has been attempted for thousands of years. Physicians raise the body temperature to between 104 and 107 degrees, either by heating the blood or by covering the body with a hot-water blanket. The treatment, lasting several weeks, has had some success reducing or slowing tumor growth, particularly in patients with melanoma or sarcomas of the limbs.

Bone-Marrow Transplant

A bone-marrow transplant, though still investigational for most cancers, is now a standard treatment option for leukemia and lymphoma. Physicians might consider a BMT, in which healthy marrow replaces diseased marrow, for a patient requiring extremely aggressive chemotherapy or irradiation. High dosages of either may severely damage or destroy the marrow, leaving the patient mortally vulnerable to infection. Leukemic patients whose marrow has been ravaged by the disease would also be appropriate candidates for the procedure.

The healthy marrow may come from one of three sources:

• In an *autologous* graft, the patient donates his own marrow when cancer cells cannot be detected microscopically; for example, when he is in remission. Harvesting the marrow is a relatively simple procedure, performed under general anesthesia. Tiny needles inserted into a bone between the hip and the spine withdraw minute amounts until approximately one quart has been collected. To ensure that the marrow is disease-free, it may be specially treated in a process called purging. Then it is frozen and reinfused intravenously days later, just like a blood transfusion.

• For an *allogeneic* transplant, the marrow is drawn from a sibling, parent, or other genetically compatible donor. Through special blood tests scientists match the patient's and donor's marrow types, which must each contain at least three of six human leukocyte antigens, or HLA. The greater the number of corresponding antigens, the less chance the patient's body will reject the graft. Close relatives, brothers and sisters in particular, generally make the most compatible donors.

• The ideal donor is an identical twin, whose HLA perfectly matches the patient's. But *syngeneic* transplants are as rare as identical twins, who account for only one birth in every two hundred seventy.

According to the National Cancer Institute, a parent or sibling has HLA-matched marrow only 30 to 40 percent of the time. And the chances of finding matching marrow from an unrelated donor are approximately one in fifteen thousand. To improve the chances of matching patients to suitable donors, the federally funded National Marrow Donor Program (3433 Broadway Street, N.E., Suite 400, Minneapolis, Minnesota 55413, 800-654-1247) conducts computer searches of transplant centers the world over.

Bone-marrow transplants can be risky. Typical complications include bleeding, liver obstruction, infection, inflammation of the mouth and gastrointestinal tract, and pneumonia. Half of all allogeneic transplant patients suffer acute graft-versus-host disease, or GVHD. As you're probably aware, in heart, liver, kidney, and other transplants, the receiver's immune system may reject the foreign organ. In a bone-marrow transplant, however, the reverse happens: the transplanted marrow identifies the body as the intruder and attacks it, most frequently in the skin, liver, and/or gastrointestinal tract. GVHD, which afflicts more older patients than young, is potentially deadly and must be treated with powerful drugs. Autologous-transplant patients, too, face serious complications, which result in death for 5 to 15 percent of them.

Presently about three thousand allogeneic bone-marrow transplants are performed each year. Physicians do not recommend the procedure lightly, as it is extremely stressful for patients and their families. Besides the physical risks and complications, at $150,000 and up—a cost rarely reimbursed by health insurers—BMTs are prohibitively expensive. In addition patients may require one or two months of hospitalization followed by another two to three months of outpatient care. According to the 1990 *International Bone Marrow Transplant Registry,* there are only 117 transplant centers nationwide, which means most patients must travel, incurring considerable added expenses.

Lastly, as with any treatment, no one can promise success. Sometimes the graft is rejected, or the donor's marrow cells fail to function adequately. For more information about bone-marrow transplants, order the National Cancer Institute's "Research Report: Bone Marrow Transplantation," available free by calling (800) 4-CANCER.

AFTERMATH

Our lives today are different in many respects since Jason's cancer. As Dr. Smithson notes, "The families that go through this often seem to grow in the process." I know that is true of everyone in our family. A child's cancer rearranges your priorities, that's for sure. I'd hate to think I would have spent my whole life worrying about whether the draperies matched the carpeting. Now I don't waste my time with trivialities.

One blessing that came from this was learning truly to appreciate my family, especially my children. I know I'll never look back in forty years and say, "I wish I'd taken more time with the kids." I also came away with a greater respect for children, their individuality and their strengths. I think as a rule we underestimate our kids, assuming that simply by virtue of being children they are emotionally and physically weak. As Jason and countless other kids we've met prove, that couldn't be farther from the truth.

In our son's case, surviving cancer has made him wise beyond his years, with a more mature perspective than most teenagers. How could it be otherwise? During a Little League play-off game Jason and Tim's team lost by one run, and on the car ride home Jason tried to cheer up his inconsolable twin.

"Boy, Tim," he said, "you really played a good game," but Tim wasn't biting. Finally Jason lost his cool. "Tim, think about it: Are you bleeding? Are you in pain? When you're forty years old, *what difference is it going to make if you lost this ball game?*"

Adam observes, "Jason's definitely changed since having cancer. Now he takes advantage of every moment, knowing that someday he might not be here. I think it's the same for our whole family."

Jason wants to be a doctor when he grows up, "so I can tell kids what having cancer is like." While our son has been blessed with the chance to pursue this dream, he will have to do so with a slight handicap.

Two years after ending treatment Jason began exhibiting signs of a minor learning disability. I thought back to the consent form I'd gratefully signed in June 1984. The two-page document clearly stated, "Radiation to the brain and/or administration of chemotherapy into the spinal fluid may produce damage to the brain." Craig and I accepted that possibility as a risk we had to take if our son was to have any future. We really didn't have much choice.

An evaluation at the Mayo Clinic confirmed that Jason had in fact suffered a degree of brain damage. According to one study 45 percent of children under age eight who received the same therapies as Jason— cranial radiation and intrathetical methotrexate—were permanently impaired intellectually to some extent.

Jason seems to have problems with reading comprehension, and we've hired a tutor to work on this. I also spend time with him on his schoolwork. We find, for example, that if I read his social-studies assignments aloud to him, he remembers the concepts more readily than if he reads it off the page.

My son also suffers occasional pain in his hips and knees, a side effect of the chemotherapy. Other potential long-term side effects that may arise anywhere from months to years after the conclusion of treatment are listed below. Whether or not your child will exhibit any of these depends on several factors, such as his age at the time of chemotherapy or radiation exposure.

• Damage to organs, including the bladder, kidneys, liver, and ovaries.
• Sterility.
• Cataracts and eye inflammation from radiation of the eye.

- Stiff joints.
- Stunted growth, from radiation of the pituitary gland, located at the base of the brain; also from the combination of chemotherapy drugs and poor nutrition during formative years.
- Impeded bone growth, especially in young children. A patient given radiation to the leg, for example, may grow up to have one leg slightly longer than the other.
- Muscle damage.
- Reduced saliva flow, or xerostomia.

Yet another possible future consequence of treatment: a second, different form of cancer. That, too, was noted in the consent form. Though the odds of such an occurrence are extremely low, the thought of a recurrence or the onset of another tumor never completely leaves you. Every ache, pain, bump, and bruise provokes worry. Not long ago my son came up behind me in the kitchen as I was washing dishes.

"Mom," he said, "I've got this weird bump. . . ."

Bump? As I spun around, heart pounding, Jason pointed to an innocent little wart on his finger. I had to laugh. *Woman,* I thought, *you've fooled yourself into thinking you're going to put this completely behind you.*

Dr. Gilchrist: "The ultimate outcome of treatment will be determined by whether or not the disease comes back. It's difficult for people to appreciate that success is measured *by the absence of failure.* That's one of the reasons why parents feel as if they're walking on eggshells all the time. When they come back with their kids to the clinic for checkups, they're often terrified."

Today Jason returns to the Mayo Clinic for an annual checkup around the time of year he was first diagnosed. Some parents find that significant anniversaries prompt anxiety. "The one thing we avoid," says Dr. Burgert, "is talking about two- or three-year survival rates. Years ago I had the experience of a family that started falling apart after two years because they thought when that two-year period was up, the bottom would fall out" and the child would relapse.

"At any point, be it one year, two years, or more, it is essential for patients to go on with their lives."

With every passing year I am plagued by fewer doubts and fears. Our lives are no longer governed by and measured against that day in June 1984. We can now look forward to other, more joyful anniversaries: of Jason's high school and college graduations, his wedding, the birth of his own children—all events that we once thought we wouldn't ever get to see.

CANCER TREATMENT, SUPPORT GROUPS, AND OTHER RESOURCES FOR THE YOUNG PATIENT AND FAMILY

The following three listings appear throughout both appendixes A and B. To avoid repetition, the addresses of their national offices are:

American Cancer Society
1599 Clifton Road, N.E., Atlanta, Georgia 30329.

Cancer Information Service (a service of the National Cancer Institute)
Office of Cancer Communications, Building 31, Room 10A24, Bethesda, Maryland 20892-3100.

Leukemia Society of America
733 Third Avenue, New York, New York 10017.

Except where indicated, all times given are local.

To Learn of Approved Cancer Programs in Your Area, Contact:

American Cancer Society
Regional offices: (800) ACS-2345, Monday through Friday, 9:00 A.M. to 5:00 P.M.
National office: (404) 320-3333.

American College of Surgeons

> 55 East Erie Street, Chicago, Illinois 60611-2797, (312) 664-4050.
> Call for referrals or request the booklet "Cancer Programs Approved."

Cancer Information Service

> (800) 4-CANCER, Monday through Friday, 9:00 A.M. to 10:00 P.M. EST.
> In Oahu, Hawaii: 524-1234; call collect from other Hawaiian islands.

For more on approved cancer programs, see Chapter Three.

To Locate a Pediatric Oncologist in Your Area, Contact:

American Cancer Society

> Regional offices: (800) ACS-2345, Monday through Friday, 9:00 A.M. to 5:00 P.M.
> National office: (404) 320-3333.

American Society of Clinical Oncology

> 435 North Michigan Avenue, Suite 1717, Chicago, Illinois 60611, (312) 644-0828.

Cancer Information Service

> (800) 4-CANCER, Monday through Friday, 9:00 A.M. to 10:00 P.M. E.S.T.
> In Oahu, Hawaii: 524-1234; call collect from other Hawaiian islands.

For more on finding a pediatric oncologist, see Chapter Three.

To Make Arrangements for a Multidisciplinary Second Opinion, Contact:

East Coast

Yale University School of Medicine
New Haven, Connecticut
(203) 785-4175

Halifax Medical Center
Daytona, Florida
(904) 254-4210

Cedars Medical Center
Miami, Florida
(305) 325-5000

Johns Hopkins Cancer Center
Baltimore, Maryland
(301) 955-8964

Norris Cotton Cancer Center
Hanover, New Hampshire
(603) 646-5505

Regional Cancer Center Lourdes
Binghamton, New York
(607) 798-5431

Montifiore Medical Center
Bronx, New York
(212) 920-4826

Roswell Park Memorial Institute
Buffalo, New York
(716) 845-3488

Mount Sinai Medical Center
New York, New York
(212) 241-6756

University of Rochester Cancer Center
Rochester, New York
(716) 275-4911

Fox Chase Cancer Center
Philadelphia, Pennsylvania
(215) 728-2986

University of Pennsylvania Cancer Center
Philadelphia, Pennsylvania
(215) 662-6364

Roger Williams Cancer Center
Providence, Rhode Island
(401) 456-2581

Middle United States

St. Vincent Cancer Center
Little Rock, Arkansas
(501) 660-3900

Loyola University
Chicago, Illinois
(312) 531-3336

Northwestern University
Chicago, Illinois
(312) 908-5284

University of Iowa Cancer Center
Iowa City, Iowa
(319) 356-3584

Comprehensive Cancer Center
Detroit, Michigan
(313) 745-8870

R. A. Bloch Cancer Management Center
Kansas City, Missouri
(816) 932-8400

Ireland Cancer Center
Cleveland, Ohio
(216) 844-8453

Ohio State University Hospital
Columbus, Ohio
(800) 4-CANCER

Thompson Cancer Survival Center
Knoxville, Tennessee
(615) 541-1757

St. Jude Children's Research Hospital
Memphis, Tennessee
(901) 522-0301

University at Texas Medical Branch at Galveston
Galveston, Texas
(409) 761-1862

University of Wisconsin Cancer Center
Madison, Wisconsin
(608) 263-8600

West Coast

Arizona Cancer Center
Tucson, Arizona
(602) 626-6372

University of California San Diego Medical Center
San Diego, California
(619) 543-6178

University of Colorado Cancer Center
Denver, Colorado
(303) 270-7235

The cancer centers in Daytona Beach, Knoxville, Little Rock, Kansas City, and Memphis offer *free* multidisciplinary second opinions.

For more on obtaining second opinions, see Chapter Three.

To Learn About Clinical Trials Being Conducted in Your Area, Contact:

Cancer Information Service
(800) 4-CANCER, Monday through Friday, 9:00 A.M. to 10:00 P.M. E.S.T.
In Oahu, Hawaii: 524-1234; call collect from other Hawaiian islands.

For more on clinical trials, see Chapter Four.

For Assistance in Matching a Patient with a Compatible Bone-Marrow Donor, Contact:

National Marrow Donor Program
3433 Broadway Street, N.E., Suite 400, Minneapolis, Minnesota 55413, (800) 654-1247.

The federally funded NMDP conducts computer searches of medical centers the world over, matching patients with allogeneic bone-marrow donors.

For more on bone-marrow transplants, see Chapter Fourteen.

To Report a Disputed Medical-Insurance Claim, Contact:

Contact the appropriate regulatory agency as listed below. The address and telephone number of each can be found in the blue-pages section of your local white pages.

TYPE OF INSURER	CONTACT
Private insurer (Blue Cross Blue Shield, Prudential, et. al.)	State Department of Insurance
Licensed health-care-services plan (Kaiser, other health-maintenance organizations)	State Department of Corporations, Division of Health-Care Services Plans
Federally qualified HMO	U.S. Department of Health and Human Services, Division of Compliance
Private employer or union self-insurance or self-financed plans	U.S. Department of Labor, Office of Pension and Welfare Benefits
Medicaid	State Department of Social Services

For more on reporting disputed medical-insurance claims, see Chapter Nine.

To Locate Cancer Support Groups in Your Area, Contact:

American Cancer Society

Regional offices: (800) ACS-2345, Monday through Friday, 9:00 A.M. to 5:00 P.M.

National office: (404) 320-3333.

In addition to offering referrals to other cancer support groups, the ACS sponsors two programs for patients and families—CanSurmount and I Can Cope.

Cancer Information Service

(800) 4-CANCER, Monday through Friday, 9:00 A.M. to 10:00 P.M. In Oahu, Hawaii: 524-1234; call collect from other Hawaiian islands.

The Candlelighters Childhood Cancer Foundation

1312 Eighteenth Street N.W., Suite 200, Washington, D.C. 20036, (800) 366-2223; (202) 659-5136 locally.

There are over three hundred Candlelighters groups for parents, patients, and siblings worldwide.

Leukemia Society of America

(800) 955-4LSA, (212) 573-8484.

The LSA sponsors thirty-two support groups nationally, all led by experienced oncology professionals.

Make Today Count

P.O. Box 6063, Kansas City, Kansas 66106, (913) 362-2866.

Approximately seventy MTC groups are scattered across the United States.

Other sources: Check with your hospital social-services department about in-house support groups and other local and regional groups.

For more on support groups, see Chapter Ten.

To Locate Bereavement Support Groups in Your Area, Contact:

The Candlelighters Childhood Cancer Foundation

1312 Eighteenth Street N.W., Suite 200, Washington, D.C. 20036, (800) 366-2223; (202) 659-5136 locally.

The Compassionate Friends
    P.O. Box 3696, Oak Brook, Illinois 60522, (708) 990-0010.

For more on bereavement, see Chapter Thirteen.

For Free Airline Transportation to Treatment Centers, Contact:
AirLifeLine
    1116 Twenty-fourth Street, Sacramento, California 95816, (916) 446-0995.

Corporate Angel Network
    Westchester County Airport, Building One, White Plains, New York 10604, (914) 328-1313.

Other sources: Your hospital social worker can inform you about additional transportation services.

For more on free airline transportation, see Chapter Seven.

For Assistance with Transportation to Doctors' Appointments, Treatment Centers, Contact:
American Cancer Society
    Regional offices: (800) ACS-2345, Monday through Friday, 9:00 A.M. to 5:00 P.M.
    National office: (404) 320-3333.
    Some ACS divisions provide drivers or reimbursement for travel expenses.

Leukemia Society of America Patient-Aid Program
    (800) 955-4LSA, (212) 573-8484.
    For patients with leukemia, preleukemia, lymphoma, or multiple myeloma, the LSA covers up to $750 of transportation costs. Check your local white pages for the chapter nearest you or call the toll-free LSA information hot line.

Other sources: Your hospital social worker can inform you about additional transportation services.

For more on assistance with transportation, see Chapter Seven.

For Nominal-Cost Shelter During Treatment Away from Home, Contact:

Ask your hospital social worker about Ronald McDonald House, a program of Ronald McDonald Children's Charities.

For more on Ronald McDonald House, see Chapter Six.

For Financial Assistance, Contact:

Leukemia Society of America Patient-Aid Program
  (800) 955-4LSA, (212) 573-8484.
  Check your local white pages for the chapter nearest you or call the toll-free LSA information hot line.

Physically Handicapped Children's Program
  Administered by your county or state Department of Health, the address and telephone number of which are listed in the blue-pages section of your local white pages.

Supplemental Security Income (SSI)
  Administered by the Social Security Administration. Visit your local Social Security office or call toll-free (800) 772-1213 weekdays from 7:00 A.M. to 7:00 P.M. EST.

Other sources: Ask your hospital social worker or financial-aid counselor about available financial aid.

For more on financial assistance, see Chapter Nine.

For Free Chemotherapy Drugs, Your Doctor Should Contact:

Adria Laboratories, Inc.
  Patient Assistance Program, P.O. Box 16529, Columbus, Ohio 43216, (614) 764-8100.
Bristol Myers Mead Johnson Pharmaceuticals
  2400 Lloyd Expressway, Evansville, Indiana 47721, (812) 429-5595.
ICI Pharmaceuticals
  P.O. Box 751, Wilmington, Delaware 19897, (800) 456-5678.

Lederle Laboratories

Building 100, North Middletown Road, Third Floor, Pearl River, New York 10965, (914) 732-2133.

Eli Lilly and Company

Lilly Corporate Center, Department MC492, Building 74-6, Indianapolis, Indiana 46285, (317) 276-2950.

Merck, Sharpe & Dohme (MSD)

West Point, Pennsylvania 19486, (215) 661-6369.

Miles, Inc., Pharmaceutical Division

400 Morgan Lane, West Haven, Connecticut 06516, (203) 937-2376.

Roche Laboratories

Professional Services Department, Nutley, New Jersey 07110, (201) 235-3071.

Other sources (for patients with either leukemia, preleukemia, lymphoma, or multiple myeloma):

Leukemia Society of America Patient-Aid Program

(800) 955-4LSA, (212) 573-8484.

Check your local white pages for the chapter nearest you or call the toll-free LSA information hot line.

For more on pharmaceutical companies' patient-assistance programs, see Chapter Nine.

For Free Loans of Hospital Beds, Wheelchairs, Commodes, Wigs, and Other Supplies, Contact:

American Cancer Society

Regional offices: (800) ACS-2345, Monday through Friday, 9:00 A.M. to 5:00 P.M.

National office: (404) 320-3333.

Other sources: Many hospitals operate free "wig banks." Check with your hospital social worker about this.

For more on wigs, hairpieces, and hair loss, see Chapter Five.

For a Free Relaxation Tape Cassette, Send an SASE Requesting "Tape" to:

Cancer Hot Line

4410 Main Street, Kansas City, Missouri 64111, (816) 932-8453.

For more on relaxation and visualization exercises, see Chapter Six.

To Locate a Trained Hypnotherapist, Contact:

American Society of Clinical Hypnosis

2200 East Devon Avenue, Suite 291, Des Plaines, Illinois 60018, (708) 297-3317.

For a list of hypnotists in your area, send an SASE, or call for a few referrals.

Society for Clinical and Experimental Hypnosis

128A Kings Park Drive, Liverpool, New York 13090, (315) 652-7299.

For a list of hypnotists in your area, send an SASE, or call for a few referrals.

For more on hypnosis, see Chapter Six.

To Locate a Trained Biofeedback Professional, Contact:

Biofeedback Society of America, 10200 West 44 Avenue, Wheat Ridge, Colorado 80033, (303) 422-8436.

For more on biofeedback, see Chapter Six.

For a Free List of Cancer Camps Nationwide, Contact:

Children's Oncology Camps of America, Inc.

Dr. Edward S. Baum, M.D., Box 30, The Children's Memorial Hospital, 2300 Children's Plaza, Chicago, Illinois 60614, (312) 880-4564.

For More on Cancer Camps, See Chapter Thirteen.

FREE CANCER-RELATED INFORMATION

RECOMMENDED FREE BOOKLETS AND HANDBOOKS

With just several toll-free phone calls, you can receive, free, these highly recommended booklets and handbooks. They are clear, concise, extremely informative, and are frequently updated.

From the National Cancer Institute:

"Chemotherapy and You/A Guide to Self-Help During Treatment"
"Diet and Nutrition: A Resource for Parents of Children with Cancer"
"Research Report: Bone Marrow Transplantation"
"Talking with Your Child About Cancer"
"Young People with Cancer: A Handbook for Parents"

On Specific Cancers

Bone Cancers
From the National Cancer Institute:

"What You Need to Know About Cancers of the Bone"
"PDQ State-of-the-Art Cancer Treatment Information/Osteosarcoma"
"PDQ State-of-the-Art Cancer Treatment Information/Ewing's Sarcoma"

Brain and Spinal-Cord Cancers
From the National Cancer Institute:

"What You Need to Know About Cancer of the Brain and Spinal Cord"
"PDQ State-of-the-Art Cancer Treatment Information/Childhood Brain Tumor"

Hodgkin's Disease and
Non-Hodgkin's Lymphomas
From the National Cancer Institute:

"Research Report: Hodgkin's Disease and the Non-Hodgkin's Lymphomas"
"What You Need to Know About Hodgkin's Disease"
"What You Need to Know About Non-Hodgkin's Lymphomas"
"PDQ State-of-the-Art Cancer Treatment Information/Childhood Hodgkin's Disease"
"PDQ State-of-the-Art Cancer Treatment Information/Childhood Non-Hodgkin's Lymphoma"

Leukemia
From the Leukemia Society of America:

"Acute Lymphocytic Leukemia"
"Chronic Myelogenous Leukemia"

From the National Cancer Institute:

"Research Report: Leukemia"
"What You Need to Know About Childhood Leukemia"
"PDQ State-of-the-Art Treatment Information/Childhood Acute Lymphocytic Leukemia"
"PDQ State-of-the-Art Treatment Information/Childhood Acute Myelogenous Leukemia"

Neuroblastoma
From the National Cancer Institute:

"PDQ State-of-the-Art Cancer Treatment Information/Neuroblastoma"

Oral Cancers
From the National Cancer Institute:

"Research Report: Oral Cancers"
"What You Need to Know About Oral Cancers"
"PDQ State-of-the-Art Treatment Information/Oral Cancers"

Retinoblastoma
From the National Cancer Institute:

"PDQ State-of-the-Art Cancer Treatment Information/Retinoblastoma"

Skin Cancers
From the National Cancer Institute:

"Research Report: Nonmelanoma Skin Cancers"
"What You Need to Know About Skin Cancer"
"PDQ State-of-the-Art Cancer Treatment Information/Skin Cancer"
"Research Report: Melanoma"
"What You Need to Know About Melanoma"
"PDQ State-of-the-Art Cancer Treatment Information/Melanoma"

From the Skin Cancer Foundation (245 Fifth Avenue, Suite 2402, New York, New York 10016, 212-725-5176):

"For Every Child Under the Sun"

Soft-Tissue Sarcomas
From the National Cancer Institute:

"Research Report: Soft Tissue Sarcomas in Adults and Children"
"PDQ State-of-the-Art Cancer Treatment Information/Childhood
   Rhabdomyosarcoma"

Wilms' Tumor
From the National Cancer Institute:

"Research Report: Adult Kidney Cancer and Wilms' Tumor"
"What You Need to Know About Kidney Cancer"
"PDQ State-of-the-Art Treatment Information/Wilms' Tumor"

For the Patient:

From the National Cancer Institute:

"Help Yourself: Tips for Teenagers with Cancer"
"Hospital Days/Treatment Ways Coloring Book"

From the Leukemia Society of America:

"Learn About Leukemia: A Coloring and Activity Book"
"What It Is That I Have, Don't Want, Didn't Ask For, Can't Give
   Back, and How I Feel About It"

From the American Cancer Society:

"What Happened to You Happened to Me"

For the Patient's Siblings:

From the National Cancer Institute:

"When Someone in Your Family Has Cancer"

From the American Cancer Society:

"When Your Brother or Sister Has Cancer"

For the Patient's Teacher(s):

From the American Cancer Society:

"Back to School: A Handbook for Teachers of Children with Cancer"

From the National Cancer Institute:

"Students with Cancer: A Resource for the Educator"

FREE* INFORMATION ABOUT AND REFERRALS TO ALTERNATIVE CANCER TREATMENT

American Cancer Society
Regional offices: (800) ACS-2345, Monday through Friday, 9:00 A.M. to 5:00 P.M.
National office: (404) 320-3333.
The ACS publishes detailed statements on some two dozen unproven methods of cancer management, available free to the public.

CanHelp
3111 Paradise Bay Road, Port Ludlow, Washington 98365, (206) 437-2291.

*CanHelp charges a fee to consult with a worldwide network of medical advisers and to prepare a report on the patient's treatment options.

Foundation for Advancement in Cancer Therapies
   P.O. Box 1242, Old Chelsea Station, New York, New York 10113,
(212) 741-2790.

International Association of Cancer Victors and Friends
   7740 West Manchester Avenue, Suite 110, Playa del Rey, California
90293, (213) 822-5032.

FOR ANSWERS TO QUESTIONS ABOUT CHILDREN'S CANCER, CALL:

American Cancer Society
   (800) ACS-2345, Monday through Friday 9:00 A.M. to 5:00 P.M.

Cancer Information Service
   (800) 4-CANCER, Monday through Friday, 9:00 A.M. to 10:00 P.M.
E.S.T.
   In Oahu, Hawaii: 524-1234; call collect from other Hawaiian islands.
   Trained staff have access to the Physicians Data Query (PDQ), a vast
computer data base on the latest advances in cancer treatment.

American Institute for Cancer Research Nutrition Hotline
   (800) 843-8114, Monday through Friday, 9:00 A.M. to 5:00 P.M. EST.
   A registered dietitian will answer your questions about diet, nutrition,
and cancer.

GLOSSARY

Anesthesiologist: A physician specializing in anesthesia. His duties include prescribing the drugs and the method of anesthesia. During surgery he either administers anesthesia personally or supervises a nurse called an anesthetist, trained in this procedure.

Angiography: An X-ray study of the blood or lymph vessels, for which patients are first injected with an opaque dye.

Antibody: A substance secreted by B-cells (a group of lymphocytes) that inactivates foreign substances, or antigens.

Benign Tumor: A noncancerous (nonmalignant) growth that does not metastasize, or spread, to other body sites.

Biological Therapy (Immunotherapy): Systemic cancer treatment (see entry) that stimulates the body's natural immune response against a specific disease.

Biopsy: Removal of cells, tissue, or fluid for microscopic examination. Biopsies are performed through incision, excision, or needle aspiration.

Blast Cell: A rapidly multiplying immature white blood cell. Normally the bone marrow contains less than 5 percent of blasts. But when a child has leukemia (see entry), these useless cells proliferate and overtake normal ones.

Bone-Marrow Aspiration: *Marrow,* the yellow or red spongy material inside large-bone cavities, manufactures blood cells (erythrocytes, leukocytes, platelets; see entries). To test its condition, doctors remove a sample from a bone in the chest, hip, spine, or leg through a suction needle. Though patients are anesthetized, a bone-marrow aspiration can cause discomfort.

Bone-Marrow Transplant: Surgical procedure that replaces a patient's destroyed marrow with healthy marrow. The marrow is harvested either from a donor or from the patient himself during remission. It is frozen and then reinfused later.

Brain Cancer: The second most common pediatric cancer, cancer of the brain and spinal cord affects mostly children ages five to ten.

Cancer: Not one but approximately one hundred diseases caused by abnormal cells that develop and divide uncontrollably, eventually crowding out and starving healthy cells. Cancerous cells can invade other tissues or organs directly, or they can migrate through the bloodstream or the lymphatic system (see entry), forming new cancers (metastases) in other parts of the body.

Carcinogen: A substance that causes cancer.

Carcinoma: Malignant invasive (see entry) growth of the epithelial cells, most often seen in cancers of the breast, uterus, intestinal tract, tongue, and skin.

Catheter: A flexible rubber, plastic, glass, or metal tube through which fluid can be injected into or withdrawn from the body.

CAT Scan (Computerized Axial Tomography): A computerized diagnostic X ray, taken cross-sectionally, which yields countless single-plane images of body tissues.

Cell-Marker Studies: A diagnostic test of biopsied bone marrow for distinguishing acute B-cell leukemia from T-cell leukemia.

Chemotherapy: Systemic cancer treatment through powerful anti-cancer drugs that are administered orally or intravenously (see entry). Often two or more medications are used in what is called combination chemotherapy.

Chromosomal Analysis: A procedure for diagnosing chronic leukemia in which harvested bone marrow is analyzed for a particular defective chromosome.

Clinical Trials: Scientific, carefully controlled studies of cancer patients to test new treatments.

Cryotherapy: Method of treating tumors whereby liquid nitrogen is sprayed on the malignancy, freezing and killing the tissue.

Dermatologist: A physician specializing in diseases of the skin.

Diagnostic: Refers to tests, procedures, devices, or substances used to detect disease.

Electrocardiography (ECG, EKG): A painless test that graphically records the heart's rhythm and other actions. Disk-shaped conductors called electrodes are attached to the body. Then an apparatus called an electrocardiograph amplifies and traces on paper the heart's minute electrical impulses.

Electrodesiccation: A method of killing remaining nonmelanoma skin-cancer cells and controlling bleeding through electrical current.

Electroencephalography (EEG): A test that records electrical activity in the brain. Electrodes are affixed to the skull with paste. Then an electroencephalograph records the electrical impulses as brain waves. Abnormal brainwave patterns suggest a possible malignancy or other disease or damage.

Endoscopy: In this procedure a flexible tubular instrument called an endoscope is inserted through the mouth, nose, or anus for viewing body cavities and hollow organs.

Erythrocytes: Red blood cells that transport oxygen to and carbon dioxide away from cells. Their red pigmentation comes from hemoglobin, an iron-rich protein.

Finger Stick: Blood-testing procedure in which a few drops of blood are taken from a fingertip that has been pricked with a sharp needle.

Gallium Scan: A type of nuclear scan (see entry) for which the patient is injected with a radioactive material called gallium-67. As it travels slowly through the body, sometimes over days, it disperses in patterns that reveal abnormalities, including cancerous lymph nodes and other tumors.

Graft: A surgical procedure in which healthy bone, skin, or other tissue replaces diseased, damaged, or amputated parts of the body.

Hematologist: A physician who specializes in the study of blood and blood-forming tissues.

Hematoma: A collection of blood or fluid that has seeped out of a vein and into an organ, space, or tissue, causing pain, swelling, or inflammation.

Hodgkin's Disease (Hodgkin's Lymphoma): The most common lymphatic-system cancer, Hodgkin's disease strikes mostly young people between ages fifteen and thirty-four. It tends to spread less extensively than non-Hodgkin's lymphomas.

Hormone Therapy: Cancer treatment by chemically supplementing or blocking hormones.

Indolent: Referring to cancers that spread slowly.

In Situ: A brief calm before the storm, when malignant cancer has yet to invade healthy tissue. In-situ tumors are generally more curable than invasive (see entry) or metastatic tumors.

Intravenous: Administering drugs, blood products, or fluids directly into a vein, either through infusion (I.V. drip) or injection (I.V. needle). Drugs can also be injected intramuscularly (into the muscle tissue), subcutaneously (just beneath the skin's surface), intraarterially (into an artery), intracavitarily (into the abdomen or the lung's pleural cavity), or intrathetically (into the spinal fluid).

Intravenous pyelography (IVP): An X-ray study of the kidneys and other abdominal organs, for which an opaque dye is injected into a vein.

Invasive Cancer: A mass of malignant cells that penetrates adjacent organ-tissue surfaces.

Laparotomy: Any abdominal surgery. When it is performed to diagnose lymphoma, the liver is sometimes biopsied and the spleen removed and examined (splenectomy). In girls, should radiation to the pelvic area be necessary, the ovaries may be elevated (ovariopexy) out of the

X-ray beam's path. For the same reason, metal clips may be implanted
to shield the left kidney.

Leukemia: The most common childhood malignancy, leukemia is
cancer of the blood and blood-producing tissues, such as the bone
marrow and the spleen. Acute lymphocytic leukemia (ALL) accounts
for 85 percent of all childhood leukemia cases. Other forms of the
disease include acute nonlymphocytic leukemias (ANLL): acute myelocytic leukemia (AML), monocytic leukemia, promyelocytic leukemia,
erythroleukemia and myelomonocytic leukemia; chronic leukemias:
chronic lymphocytic leukemia (CLL), and hairy-cell leukemia, and
chronic myelogenous leukemia (CML).

Leukocytes: Mature white blood cells that help protect the body
against infection. There are three main types: granulocytes, lymphocytes, and monocytes.

Localized Cancer: A malignancy found only in the original (primary) site.

Lumbar Puncture (Spinal Tap): Diagnostic procedure in which
spinal fluid is withdrawn from (or chemotherapeutic or anesthetic drugs
are injected into) the lower spinal area with a needle.

Lymph: A clear yellowish fluid consisting primarily of white blood
cells called lymphocytes, lymph travels through the lymphatic system to
bathe body tissues and help combat infection.

Lymphangiography: An X-ray study in which the lymph nodes (see
entry) and vessels are outlined to reveal any abnormalities. Patients are
injected with a contrast dye beforehand.

Lymphatic System: Part of the body's circulatory system, the lymphatic system is comprised of a network of vessels that transport lymph
throughout the body. Lymph nodes (see entry), the spleen, the thymus
gland, the tonsils, and the bone marrow also make up this disease- and
infection-fighting system.

Lymphoma: Cancer of the lymphatic system. There are at least ten
types of non-Hodgkin's lymphomas. Indolent lymphomas develop
slowly, while aggressive types spread rapidly and can be quickly fatal.

Non-Hodgkin's lymphomas are most often found in children ages five to fourteen.

Lymph Nodes: Bean-shaped organs that filter bacteria, viruses, dead cells, and other harmful agents from the lymphatic system.

Magnetic Resonance Imaging (MRI): A relatively new, noninvasive imaging technique, similar to a CAT scan, which creates cross-sectional pictures of the body by means of a powerful magnet linked to a computer.

Malignant Tumor: A cancerous tumor capable of metastasizing.

Metastasis: The process by which a colony of malignant cells separates from the primary site and travels to another not adjacent or connected to it.

Micrometastasis: The migration of microscopic, undetectable, cancer cells.

Myeloma: Cancer that originates in the bone marrow, in the antibody-secreting plasma cells.

Neoplasm: Any new, uncontrolled growth of abnormal tissue, or tumor. It can be benign or malignant.

Nephrotomography: A three-dimensional X-ray study of the kidney.

Neuroblastoma: A common pediatric cancer that originates in the nervous system, neuroblastoma strikes mainly children under age five. More than half of neuroblastomas develop in the abdomen's adrenal glands, but the disease can also arise in the eyes, neck, chest, and pelvis.

Neurologist: A physician specializing in diseases of the brain, nerves, and nervous system.

Nuclear Scans (Radioisotope Studies): Children either swallow or are injected with a harmless radioactive material, which electronic devices then track through the body to help physicians determine whether or not organs such as the kidneys, liver, and brain are functioning properly. These scans actually expose patients to less radiation than regular X rays.

Oncologist: A physician who specializes in the study of cancer (oncology).

Ophthamologist: A physician specializing in diseases of the eye.

Oral Cancer: Rare in children, oral cancer develops in the oral cavity; most often the lips, the cheek lining, the gums, or the floor of the mouth. The most common oral cancer, squamous-cell carcinoma, develops in the thin cells lining the oral cavity and the skin. Basal-cell carcinoma arises in the basal cells in the skin's deepest layers, while melanoma originates in the melanocytes, the cells that produce skin pigment.

Pathologist: A doctor specializing in identifying diseases through microscopic study.

Photocoagulation: Method of treating certain small tumors by destroying with heat from a light beam the blood vessels that feed them.

Platelets: One of the blood's components, these disk-shaped cells prevent profuse bleeding, or hemorrhaging, by coagulating and forming clots.

Prognosis: A prediction of a disease's likely outcome; an assessment of the patient's chances for recovery.

Protocol: A standardized, detailed treatment program for a particular type of cancer.

Rad: *R*adiation *A*bsorbed *D*ose. A unit of measurement of the absorbed dose of radiation.

Radiation Therapy: Treatment of disease by means of ionizing radiation from X-ray machines, cobalt, radium, and other sources. Administered by a radiotherapist.

Radiologist: A physician specially trained in radiology, the science of interpreting medical X rays.

Regression: A return to a previous state. In cancer, regression occurs when, for example, tumors shrink or disappear and/or disease otherwise subsides.

Relapse: Cancer's reappearance after a period during which its symptoms had abated or vanished.

Remission: Temporary or permanent condition in which no cancer is detected, though cancerous cells may remain in the body. Patients are then said to be "in remission."

Retinoblastoma: A relatively rare congenital cancer of the eye that generally afflicts children under age four and in one of three cases is bilateral; that is, involving both eyes.

Sarcoma: A malignant tumor that originates in bones, cartilage, muscle, blood vessels, or lymphoid tissue. Sarcomas often metastasize by way of the lymph system and grow rapidly. Among those prevalent in children are osteosarcoma (bone), rhabdomyosarcoma (soft tissue), and Ewing's sarcoma, an aggressive cancer that develops in bones' marrow spaces. Chondrosarcoma, rare in children, attacks the cartilage.

Selective Renal Arteriography: An X-ray study of the kidneys' veins and arteries, for which an opaque substance is first injected into the bloodstream.

Skin Cancer: Caused mainly by the sun's ultraviolet rays. Squamous-cell carcinoma develops in the thin cells that line the oral cavity and the skin; basal-cell carcinoma, in the round basal cells in the skin's deepest layers, or dermis; and melanoma, in the melanocytes, the cells that produce skin pigment.

Staging: A classification system for identifying the extent of disease.

Systemic Treatment: Cancer therapy that affects cells throughout the body, such as chemotherapy.

Topical Chemotherapy: Method of treating nonmelanoma skin cancer with an anticancer cream or lotion to the affected area.

Ultrasonography: An imaging method that uses the reflections, or echoes, of ultrasonic waves on body tissue to create "pictures."

Wilms' Tumor: This rapidly developing malignant tumor originates in the kidneys and affects only children, from infancy to age fifteen.

Once considered fatal, Wilms' tumor is now one of the most curable forms of pediatric cancer.

X rays: High-energy electromagnetic radiation used in low dosages to "photograph" the inner body and in high dosages to treat cancer.

ABOUT THE AUTHORS

GERALYN and CRAIG GAES and their four children were the subject of the 1989 Academy Award–winning documentary *You Don't Have to Die*, about their son Jason's struggle against Burkitt's lymphoma. The Gaeses frequently speak around the country on behalf of cancer-related organizations such as Ronald McDonald Children's Charities, the American Cancer Society, and the Candlelighters Childhood Cancer Foundation. They live in St. Joseph, Missouri.

PHILIP BASHE has written or cowritten the books *Teenage Idol, Travelin' Man, That's Not All Folks!, When Saying No Isn't Enough: How to Keep the Children You Love Off Drugs, Dee Snider's Teenage Survival Guide, Heavy Metal Thunder,* the *Rolling Stone Rock Almanac,* and the forthcoming *Dogdays: The New York Yankees' Fall from Grace and Eventual Redemption.* A former magazine editor-writer and radio announcer, he is a member of the Author's Guild. Bashe resides with his wife, author Patricia Romanowski, and son, Justin, in Baldwin, New York.